Mental Health, Diabetes and Endocrinology

Mental Health, Diabetes and Endocrinology

Edited by

Anne M. Doherty
University College Dublin

Aoife M. Egan
Division of Endocrinology and Metabolism, Mayo Clinic

Seán F. Dinneen
School of Medicine, National University of Ireland Galway

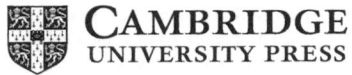
CAMBRIDGE
UNIVERSITY PRESS

CAMBRIDGE
UNIVERSITY PRESS

University Printing House, Cambridge CB2 8BS, United Kingdom

One Liberty Plaza, 20th Floor, New York, NY 10006, USA

477 Williamstown Road, Port Melbourne, VIC 3207, Australia

314–321, 3rd Floor, Plot 3, Splendor Forum, Jasola District Centre, New Delhi – 110025, India

103 Penang Road, #05–06/07, Visioncrest Commercial, Singapore 238467

Cambridge University Press is part of the University of Cambridge.

It furthers the University's mission by disseminating knowledge in the pursuit of education, learning, and research at the highest international levels of excellence.

www.cambridge.org
Information on this title: www.cambridge.org/9781911623618
DOI: 10.1017/9781911623625

© Cambridge University Press 2021

First published 2021

Printed in the United Kingdom by TJ Books Limited, Padstow Cornwal

A catalogue record for this publication is available from the British Library.

Library of Congress Cataloging-in-Publication Data
Names: Doherty, Anne M., 1981– editor. | Egan, Aoife M., 1983– editor. | Dinneen, Seán F., editor.
Title: Mental health, diabetes and endocrinology / edited by Anne M. Doherty, Aoife M. Egan, Seán F. Dinneen.
Description: Cambridge, United Kingdom ; New York, NY : Cambridge University Press, 2021. | Includes bibliographical references and index.
Identifiers: LCCN 2021019478 (print) | LCCN 2021019479 (ebook) | ISBN 9781911623618 (paperback) | ISBN 9781911623625 (epub)
Subjects: MESH: Mental Disorders--complications | Endocrine System Diseases--complications | Diabetes Complications
Classification: LCC RC454 (print) | LCC RC454 (ebook) | NLM WM 140 | DDC 616.89--dc23
LC record available at https://lccn.loc.gov/2021019478
LC ebook record available at https://lccn.loc.gov/2021019479

ISBN 978-1-911-62361-8 Paperback

••

Contents

Contributors

Mary Davoren: Consultant Forensic Psychiatrist, Central Mental Hospital; Senior Lecturer in Psychiatry, Trinity College Dublin.
Prior to her appointment to the Central Mental Hospital, Dundrum, in 2019, Dr Mary Davoren was a consultant forensic psychiatrist in Broadmoor Hospital, the high secure facility for Greater London and the south of England, where she was the High Secure Research Lead, the Responsible Clinician on the Broadmoor Personality Disorder Pathway and an academic coordinator for the Broadmoor Seminar Conference Series. Prior to that appointment, she completed an Academic Clinical Fellowship at the Violence Prevention Research Unit, Queen Mary University of London, an affiliated centre of the World Health Organization (WHO) Violence Prevention Alliance, and an MD in research at Trinity College Dublin. Her main research interests include the systematic use of routine outcome measures in secure forensic mental health settings and the physical health of patients in secure forensic hospitals and prisons.

Diana S. Dean: Consultant and Associate Professor of Medicine, Division of Endocrinology and Metabolism at Mayo Clinic.
Dr Diana S. Dean attended the University of the South in Sewanee, Tennessee, where she graduated cum laude with a BA degree in biology. She received her MD degree from the University of Alabama School of Medicine in Birmingham, Alabama. She pursued training in internal medicine and endocrinology at Mayo Clinic and became a member of the faculty in 2002. Her main clinical interests include benign and malignant disorders of the thyroid gland and ultrasound-guided fine-needle aspiration of thyroid nodules. Dr Dean combines her clinical interests with a strong passion for education and speaking.

Seán F. Dinneen: Consultant Endocrinologist, Galway University Hospitals; Professor of Diabetic Medicine, School of Medicine, National University of Ireland Galway; National Lead, Diabetes Clinical Programme (Ireland).
Professor Seán F. Dinneen graduated from University College Cork Medical School. After postgraduate training and work in the USA (Mayo Clinic), Canada (McMaster University) and the UK (Addenbrooke's Hospital), he returned to Ireland as an academic endocrinologist. He served as head of the School of Medicine from 2013 to 2016. In 2016, he was appointed National Lead for the Diabetes Clinical Programme (Ireland). His interests include self-management education and support for people living with diabetes, developing community-based diabetes care and the diabetic foot. He is a regional editor for *Diabetic Medicine* and Clinical Lead for Schwartz Rounds in Galway University Hospitals.

Anne M. Doherty: Associate Professor of Psychiatry, University College Dublin; Consultant Liaison Psychiatrist, Mater Misericordiae University Hospital Dublin; Chair Faculty of Liaison Psychiatry, College of Psychiatrists of Ireland.
Prior to her 2020 appointment to University College Dublin, Dr Anne M. Doherty was a consultant in liaison psychiatry at Galway University Hospitals. From 2012 to 2016, she was a consultant liaison psychiatrist at King's College

Hospital, London, leading the 3 Dimensions of Care for Diabetes service, an award-winning (BMJ Team of the Year Award 2014, NHS Innovation Challenge Prize 2015) multidisciplinary team for people with poorly controlled diabetes. She contributed to the Joint British Diabetes Societies for Inpatient Care (JBDS–IP) and Royal College of Psychiatrists (RCPsych) Guidelines on Management of Diabetes in Adults and Children with Psychiatric Disorders (2017). Her research interests include adjustment disorders in acute hospitals (the subject of her research MD), suicidality and the interface between psychiatry and other medical conditions.

Aoife M. Egan: Consultant and Assistant Professor of Medicine, Division of Endocrinology and Metabolism at Mayo Clinic.
Dr Aoife M. Egan graduated from the School of Medicine at the National University of Ireland Galway (MB BCh BAO). She then completed training in general internal medicine followed by speciality training in endocrinology, which incorporated a PhD in medicine. Dr Egan subsequently pursued further fellowship training at Mayo Clinic and was appointed to her current position in 2020. Her research interests include the pathophysiology and management of pre-gestational and gestational diabetes and the long-term risk of type 2 diabetes in women with gestational diabetes.

Eimear Morrissey: Health Psychologist and Postdoctoral Researcher, National University of Ireland Galway.
Dr Eimear Morrissey graduated from the National University of Ireland Galway in 2018 with a PhD in health psychology. She is currently managing 'D1 Now', a research project that aims to develop an intervention to support the self-management of young adults living with type 1 diabetes. She has more than 20 publications, including journal articles, book chapters and policy briefs. She is actively involved in the wider health psychology community, having served as the treasurer for CREATE (an early career research network within the European Health Psychology Society) for two years, and she is currently Public Relations Officer of the Psychological Society of Ireland Division of Health Psychology. Dr Morrissey's research interests include the self-management of chronic disease, treatment adherence, digital interventions and behaviour change science.

Todd B. Nippoldt: Consultant Endocrinologist and Associate Professor of Medicine, Division of Endocrinology and Metabolism at Mayo Clinic.
Dr Todd B. Nippoldt attended the Institute of Technology, University of Minnesota, where he graduated with a BMechE degree (mechanical engineering). He received his MD degree from the Mayo Clinic Alix School of Medicine in 1982. He pursued training in internal medicine and endocrinology at Mayo Clinic and completed a fellowship in Endocrinology and Metabolism at the University of Michigan in 1988. His main clinical and research interests include transgender health, reproductive endocrinology and pituitary disorders. He is Medical Director at Mayo Clinic's Transgender Intersex Specialty Care Clinic.

Preface

We were inspired to write this book by our experience in clinical practice and the specific challenges of managing comorbid mental disorders and endocrine conditions, and in recognition of the impact that stress, distress and mental illness can have on the management of physical illness, especially in endocrinology.

Mental Health, Diabetes and Endocrinology will examine key clinical areas of overlap between the two specialities, studying the main topics of interest and common challenges. It is written for clinicians and will draw together the most relevant developments from the literature and clinical practice. This book will pay specific attention to the main areas where clinical conundrums and treatment challenges arise across endocrinology, psychiatry and primary care. Common challenges in this area include depression, which can impact on a person's ability to self-care and adhere to treatment, with consequences for their morbidity and mortality; 'diabulimia', or comorbid diabetes and eating disorder, which is associated with high mortality rates; obesity and associated mental disorders; cognitive impairment and mental capacity; antipsychotic medications and their endocrine and metabolic sequelae; and specific setting-related concerns.

We hope that *Mental Health, Diabetes and Endocrinology* will be a useful resource regarding overlapping conditions across the specialities and a valuable reference for all healthcare professionals who encounter these issues.

We considered taking a more traditional approach to this book by systematically proceeding through each of the major endocrine disorders and addressing the common psychiatric comorbidities. However, it seemed more useful to focus on those areas that are associated with the most complex clinical scenarios. We hope that this approach will prove useful to readers regarding the common conundrums that arise in clinical practice.

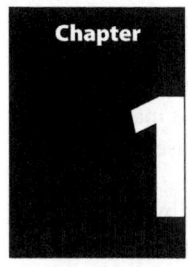

Chapter 1

An Introduction to Psychiatry in Endocrinology

Anne M. Doherty and Seán F. Dinneen

Introduction

Modern developments in research and services have demonstrated the need for better integration of mental and physical healthcare in various areas of medicine, including endocrinology. Years of research have shown the importance of the stress response and the hypothalamic–pituitary–end organ axes in the aetiology of depression and many common mental disorders.

In the nineteenth century, the eminent London psychiatrist Henry Maudsley noted that 'diabetes is a disease which often shows itself in families in which insanity prevails'. In more recent years, the evolving literature on the topic has not only made it evident that diabetes is more common among people who have mental disorders but also shown that mental disorders are more common among people living with diabetes, thyroid disease and obesity. Depression, for example, is twice as common in people with diabetes compared with the general population. Diabetes is also diagnosed at a disproportionately higher rate among patients with a diagnosis of a psychotic disorder. Overall, there is a high proportion of mental disorders in any population of people with diabetes, and where these comorbidities are present, they contribute to the mortality gap between people with major mental illness and the general population.

In recent decades, research efforts have moved on from demonstrating the association between mental disorders and endocrinology conditions to developing tailored treatments for patients with these comorbidities. Research in the past decade has suggested that integrated care may be a key approach to the clinical management of comorbid diabetes and depression, and further research is likely to show that this may be generalisable to other mental and physical comorbidities. In many clinical centres, especially in the areas of obesity and gender medicine, endocrinologists and psychiatrists, psychologists or other mental health specialists work together to provide care that integrates the needs of the body and the mind.

Patients with schizophrenia and other psychotic disorders are at greater risk of developing disorders such as metabolic syndrome, prediabetes and diabetes. It remains unclear whether this relates in some way to the nature of psychosis, but we know that atypical antipsychotics certainly contribute to a significant degree, with olanzapine and clozapine having a particularly large impact on metabolic syndromes (see Chapter 3). Other (typical and atypical) neuroleptic medications have central effects on the release of hormones such as prolactin.

The aetiology of depression is considered to be multifactorial, with various factors, including genetics, life events and stress, contributing to the development of depressive symptoms via the hypothalamic–pituitary–adrenal (HPA) axis, and there are also newer theories on this matter regarding inflammation and the HPA–gut axis. There is some evidence that inflammation may represent a shared pathway for depression and type 2 diabetes (1). Hyperthyroidism can result in symptoms of depression and anxiety; these are discussed in more detail in Chapter 6. Furthermore, an Addisonian crisis may present in a very similar way to an agitated depression (i.e. depression with increased rather than diminished psychomotor activity).

The epidemiology of mental and endocrine disorders is complicated by the complex relationship between these conditions. The larger psychiatric epidemiological studies have not examined endocrinological comorbidity. We know that people with depression have a higher risk of being diagnosed with diabetes. Likewise, there are high rates of comorbidity between many mental disorders and type 1 diabetes, type 2 diabetes, obesity, thyroid disease, parathyroid disease, Addison's disease, Cushing's syndrome, etc. (2–7). Some neuropsychiatric symptoms may be explained entirely by comorbid endocrine conditions and may resolve when these are treated.

Clinical Needs of Specific Groups

Throughout this book, we discuss the needs of specific groups of patients who have comorbidities with endocrine and mental disorders. Those patients who are seen predominantly in a medical setting will often receive their psychiatry input from a liaison psychiatry or psychological medicine team. However, those who have a mental disorder as their predominant illness with secondary metabolic syndrome due to either the mental disorder or the treatment of it are likely to be treated chiefly in secondary care mental health settings with management of endocrine comorbidities by specialists in endocrinology or primary care medicine. Therefore, it is important that both sets of professionals have a good understanding of the other side of the comorbidity so that they can best manage and integrate patient care. There are specific complexities that relate to older patients and those with cognitive impairment. Furthermore, patients with the combination of diabetes and eating disorder deserve special attention because of the significant risk of insulin omission (particularly in type 1 diabetes) and the associated poor outcomes. Throughout this book, we discuss service delivery considerations relating to how patients with these combinations of complex comorbidities are best managed and what services need to do in order to meet patients' needs and to optimise their overall treatment and care.

Overview of Clinical Developments in Endocrinology

In the 1990s, with an increasing recognition of endocrinopathies occurring in patients post organ transplantation, many medical centres developed joint endocrine–transplant clinics to encourage a multidisciplinary approach to metabolic disorders, bone loss and issues with fertility in this cohort of patients. More recently, the introduction of the checkpoint inhibitor class of cancer immunotherapies has resulted in a plethora of endocrinopathies being recognised as side effects of these agents, and endocrinologists and medical oncologists are increasingly working together to tackle the challenging clinical issues that can arise when, for example, patients undergoing cancer treatment develop Addison's disease, thyroid disorders or type 1 diabetes. This pattern of endocrinologists working closely with specialists from other disciplines has not been the norm in the interface between endocrine disorders and psychiatric conditions. Gender dysphoria and bariatric medicine may be the exceptions, as careful assessment of a patient's premorbid psychological state is recognised as a key determinant of long-term success with the planned (gender transition/affirmation or weight loss) intervention. These issues are discussed in greater detail in Chapters 10 and 11.

Type 2 diabetes is by far the most common endocrine disorder encountered by psychiatrists. While a comprehensive overview of the management of type 2 diabetes is beyond the scope of this book, it is important that practising psychiatrists have some familiarity with recent developments in diabetology, which include the following:

(1) A recognition of the importance of programmes of self-management (behaviour change) education for patients newly diagnosed with type 2 diabetes or even prior to diagnosis (in which case these are referred to as diabetes prevention programmes).

(2) The introduction of new classes of oral (SGLT-2 inhibitor) and injectable (GLP-1 receptor agonist) therapies that have the potential to reduce cardiovascular events as well as lower plasma glucose.

(3) A rise in population-wide screening programmes for diabetic complications, with retinal and foot screening programmes now recognised as having essential roles in reducing vision loss and limb loss from diabetes.

Psychiatry in the General Hospital

The speciality of liaison psychiatry or psychological medicine emerged in the latter decades of the twentieth century and relates to the expert management of mental health problems in the acute hospital setting. Liaison psychiatry was first recognised as a faculty of the Royal College of Psychiatrists in the UK in 1997. It has been recognised as a sub-speciality of the American Psychiatric Association since 2004, and in the USA it is known as psychosomatic medicine or consultation–liaison psychiatry.

A liaison psychiatry team will usually include psychiatrists who are specialists in the management of mental health problems in the context of physical illness and working in physical health settings, as well as junior doctors or psychiatrists in training; specialist mental health nurses; clinical or health psychologists with an interest in the overlap between mental and physical health; and perhaps social workers, occupational therapists and pharmacists.

A properly resourced liaison psychiatry team will provide a comprehensive service to patients in the acute hospital setting who may have mental health needs alongside their physical health needs. They will ideally be adequately resourced not only to see patients presenting to the emergency department with acute psychiatric illness, including self-harm and psychosis, but also to provide assessment of and treat patients on medical and surgical wards who require mental healthcare alongside their acute medical or surgical healthcare needs. Liaison psychiatry services may also run outpatient clinics for patients who have comorbid mental and physical health problems. These will include people with functional conditions (or 'medically unexplained' symptoms) or anxiety that presents with predominately physical symptoms, as well as chronic conditions such as diabetes, where the comorbid mental illness is creating a barrier to adequate self-management.

In endocrinology, the liaison psychiatrist or liaison psychiatry team can work with an endocrinology team to improve the outcomes for their patients through integration of their mental and physical healthcare. There are specific areas where this is valuable – often these are scenarios or conditions that are not considered to be related to psychiatry by non-specialists. Such an example is the assessment of people presenting with recurrent unexplained episodes of diabetic ketoacidosis, which is a red flag for psychiatric assessment (see Chapter 9). In diabetes, for example, patients may develop a number of psychological barriers to good diabetes management in addition to having a comorbid mental disorder. Such psychological barriers may include a fear of hypoglycaemia; a fear of needles; weight and shape concerns; or even a disabling fear of developing the end-stage complications of diabetes, precipitating a state of denial. Once these barriers are identified, they can become targets for treatment, such as a cognitive behavioural therapy (CBT) model of treatment. CBT models focus on examining the person's thoughts, feelings, physical sensations and behaviours, considering how they interact with one another and working with the patient to find a more adaptive way of relating to their diabetes.

Innovative Models of Service Delivery

Internationally, there are a number of key examples of embedded mental health services in endocrinology teams, such as those at King's College Hospital in London. Often these endocrinology-specific mental health services are integrated with one aspect of endocrinology care, such as diabetes or bariatric medicine or in gender clinics. There are also service models such as the TEAMcare delivery model developed by the late Wayne Katon and colleagues in the USA.

TEAMcare is a novel initiative that was developed in Seattle in the early twenty-first century. Dr Katon and colleagues devised a treatment programme for patients who had comorbid depression along with diabetes or heart failure. This programme was delivered in primary care predominantly by a mental health nurse who provided psychological therapies mainly based on a CBT model. This nurse had access to a psychiatrist if psychotropic medication was required, and the primary care physician provided the cardiac and diabetes care. This service model was found to be effective both clinically and in terms of cost-effectiveness (8, 9). A number of papers from this group have demonstrated that integrating mental and physical healthcare in this way is successful in terms of both patients' health and the efficiency of the healthcare organisation (10, 11).

In south London, Khalida Ismail and her group have delivered a number of complex interventions in both research and clinical settings. One of these was the A Diabetes and Psychological Therapies (ADaPT) study, which was a randomised controlled trial (RCT) of CBT versus motivational interviewing (MI) or a combination thereof delivered by diabetes nurses. The ADaPT study found that a combination of CBT and MI was most effective at improving glycaemic control (12, 13). The D-6 study, which also randomised basic CBT and MI to support the self-management of patients with type 2 diabetes, did not find any improvements associated with these interventions (14). Ismail's south London group developed the experimental 3 Dimensions of Care for Diabetes (3DFD) programme, which was an intensive intervention focusing on patients with poorly controlled diabetes (HbA1c > 75 mmol/mol) and offering patients in this group a complex intervention. This intervention was tailored to the patients' needs and included input from psychiatry, psychology and social support, with the aim of identifying and meeting the needs of the patients, especially those presenting with barriers to the optimal management of their diabetes. This non-randomised study reported significant improvements in the intervention group compared with a comparison group, with an improvement in mean HbA1c of 16 mmol/mol in the intervention group, as well as improvements in blood pressure, weight, lipids and psychological measures. Unfortunately, due to the complex and expensive nature of the intervention, it was no cheaper than regular care, but it is worth noting that the analyses did not factor in the impact of the observed reduction in HbA1c of 16 mmol/mol, which is typically associated with significant reductions in a patient's risk of developing macrovascular and microvascular complications, and therefore may be associated with long-term reductions in the cost of care (15, 16).

A systematic review of collaborative care by Atlantis et al. concluded that collaborative care significantly improved depression and glycaemic control in individuals with diabetes and depression. However, the overall weighted mean difference was small, the meaning of collaborative care varied widely and most of the studies had limited generalisability outside of the USA (17). A cluster RCT of collaborative care in a UK primary care setting found a modest improvement in depressive symptoms at four months but did not examine glycaemic control or any physical health outcomes (18). Subsequent analysis showed that it was a cost-effective intervention based on improvements in quality-adjusted life-years (19).

Similar models of care have been implemented in Sweden and the UK for older patients with depression alongside physical multi-morbidity, and these models have been found to be acceptable to patients and practical to implement (20, 21).

Conclusion

Comorbidities of endocrine and psychiatric conditions are common. Both conditions need to be treated, and the evidence is growing that an integrated approach may yield better outcomes, but this requires an additional level of expertise in working across the domains, and often personal flexibility in teams that are reaching out beyond their usual areas of practice. Where collaborative care or integrated care systems or interventions have been implemented, they have shown improved outcomes across the domains, but apart from in bariatric medicine and gender medicine, these are not yet considered essential components of treatment. There is a need for more research into the management of complex comorbidities in order to build on this evidence base further and to promote fully integrated care for people with these interlocking comorbidities.

References

1 Moulton CD, Pickup JC, Rokakis AS, Amiel SA, Ismail K, Stahl D. The prospective association between inflammation and depressive symptoms in type 2 diabetes stratified by sex. *Diabetes Care*. 2019; 42(10): 1865–72.

2 Luppino FS, de Wit LM, Bouvy PF, Stijnen T, Cuijpers P, Penninx BW, et al. Overweight, obesity, and depression: a systematic review and meta-analysis of longitudinal studies. *Arch Gen Psychiatry*. 2010; 67(3): 220–9.

3 Barnard KD, Skinner TC, Peveler R. The prevalence of co-morbid depression in adults with type 1 diabetes: systematic literature review. *Diabet Med*. 2006; 23(4): 445–8.

4 Ali S, Stone MA, Peters JL, Davies MJ, Khunti K. The prevalence of co-morbid depression in adults with type 2 diabetes: a systematic review and meta-analysis. *Diabet Med*. 2006; 23(11): 1165–73.

5 Suliburk JW, Perrier ND. Primary hyperparathyroidism. *Oncologist*. 2007; 12 (6): 644–53.

6 Siegmann EM, Muller HHO, Luecke C, Philipsen A, Kornhuber J, Gromer TW. Association of depression and anxiety disorders with autoimmune thyroiditis: a systematic review and meta-analysis. *JAMA Psychiatry*. 2018; 75(6): 577–84.

7 Musselman DL, Nemeroff CB. Depression and endocrine disorders: focus on the thyroid and adrenal system. *Br J Psychiatry Suppl*. 1996; (30): 123–8.

8   Katon WJ, Lin EH, Von Korff M, Ciechanowski P, Ludman EJ, Young B, et al. Collaborative care for patients with depression and chronic illnesses. *N Engl J Med*. 2010; 363(27): 2611–20.

9   Katon W, Russo J, Lin EH, Schmittdiel J, Ciechanowski P, Ludman E, et al. Cost-effectiveness of a multicondition collaborative care intervention: a randomized controlled trial. *Arch Gen Psychiatry*. 2012; 69(5): 506–14.

10 McGregor M, Lin EH, Katon WJ. TEAMcare: an integrated multicondition collaborative care program for chronic illnesses and depression. *J Ambul Care Manage*. 2011; 34(2): 152–62.

11 Lin EH, Von Korff M, Ciechanowski P, Peterson D, Ludman EJ, Rutter CM, et al. Treatment adjustment and medication adherence for complex patients with diabetes, heart disease, and depression: a randomized controlled trial. *Ann Fam Med*. 2012; 10(1): 6–14.

12 Ismail K, Maissi E, Thomas S, Chalder T, Schmidt U, Bartlett J, et al. A randomised controlled trial of cognitive behaviour therapy and motivational interviewing for people with type 1 diabetes mellitus with persistent sub-optimal glycaemic control: a Diabetes and Psychological Therapies (ADaPT) study. *Health Technol Assess*. 2010; 14(22): 1–101, iii–iv.

13 Ridge K, Bartlett J, Cheah Y, Thomas S, Lawrence-Smith G, Winkley K, et al. Do the effects of psychological treatments on improving glycemic control in type 1 diabetes persist over time? A long-term follow-up of a randomized controlled trial. *Psychosom Med*. 2012; 74(3): 319–23.

14 Ismail K, Winkley K, de Zoysa N, Patel A, Heslin M, Graves H, et al. Nurse-led psychological intervention for type 2 diabetes: a cluster randomised controlled trial (Diabetes-6 study) in primary care. *Br J Gen Pract*. 2018; 68(673): e531–40.

15 Ismail K, Stewart K, Ridge K, Britneff E, Freudenthal R, Stahl D, et al. A pilot study of an integrated mental health, social and medical model for diabetes care in an inner-city setting: Three Dimensions for Diabetes (3DFD). *Diabet Med*. 2020; 37 (10): 1658–68.

16 Doherty AM, Gayle C, Morgan-Jones R, Archer N, Laura L, Ismail K, et al. Improving quality of diabetes care by integrating psychological and social care for poorly controlled diabetes: 3 Dimensions of Care for Diabetes. *Int J Psychiatry Med*. 2016; 51(1): 3–15.

17 Atlantis E, Fahey P, Foster J. Collaborative care for comorbid depression and diabetes: a systematic review and meta-analysis. *BMJ Open*. 2014; 4(4): e004706.

18 Coventry P, Lovell K, Dickens C, Bower P, Chew-Graham C, McElvenny D, et al. Integrated primary care for patients with mental and physical multimorbidity: cluster randomised controlled trial of collaborative care for patients with depression comorbid with diabetes or cardiovascular disease. *BMJ*. 2015; 350: h638.

19 Camacho EM, Davies LM, Hann M, Small N, Bower P, Chew-Graham C, et al. Long-term clinical and cost-effectiveness of collaborative care (versus usual care) for people with mental–physical multimorbidity: cluster-randomised trial. *Br J Psychiatry*. 2018; 213(2): 456–63.

20 Augustsson P, Holst A, Svenningsson I, Petersson EL, Björkelund C, Björk Brämberg E. Implementation of care managers for patients with depression: a cross-sectional study in Swedish primary care. *BMJ Open*. 2020; 10(5): e035629.

21 Taylor AK, Gilbody S, Bosanquet K, Overend K, Bailey D, Foster D, et al. How should we implement collaborative care for older people with depression? A qualitative study using normalisation process theory within the CASPER plus trial. *BMC Fam Pract*. 2018; 19(1): 116.

Depression across Endocrine Disorders

Anne M. Doherty and Seán F. Dinneen

Introduction

Depression is a common mental illness that is receiving increasing clinical, academic and even political attention. The World Health Organization (WHO) stated in its report of 2004 that depression is one of the most significant health challenges of the twenty-first century in terms of its effect on disability and loss of function, and ranked it as the third leading cause of burden of disease worldwide as measured by disease-adjusted life-years (1). It is the leading cause of disease burden in the Americas and is projected to be the leading cause worldwide by 2030. It is the subject of thousands of books and hundreds of thousands of peer-reviewed scientific articles – entering the search term into PubMed alone yields over 550,000 articles.

In addition to being an important condition in its own right, it is increasingly being recognised as a condition that has a significant effect on recovery and even mortality when comorbid with physical illness (2, 3). Comorbid mental disorders with endocrine conditions may present challenges both for the patient and their healthcare providers. The evidence for effective joint interventions is at an early stage, and individuals with psychiatric disorders often experience inequalities in accessing routine physical healthcare.

Epidemiology of Depression and Impact on Physical Health

Depression is a common disorder that is underdiagnosed and undertreated despite increasing public awareness, especially in the developed world. It is ranked by the WHO as one of the leading causes of morbidity worldwide (4). It may present at any point along the lifespan, with incidence and prevalence highest in the early 20s (5). The prevalence of depression in the general population is 5%, and patients with a medical condition are at least twice as likely to have a comorbid depression compared to the general population (6, 7).

Lifetime prevalence rates have been estimated quite differently depending on the measures used: in the United States Epidemiological Catchment Area (ECA) study it was estimated as 4.4% (8), in the National Co-morbidity Study (NCS) (9) it was estimated as 17.1% and in the Virginia Twin Study it was as high as 30.0% (10).

Both type 1 and type 2 diabetes are associated with at least double the risk of depression compared to the general public. On meta-analysis, depression is present in 12.0% of patients with type 1 diabetes and 17.6% of patients with type 2 diabetes (11, 12). A prospective case–control study found depression in 17% of people with primary hyperparathyroidism compared with 7% of controls (13). The odds ratio (OR) for coexisting depression in autoimmune thyroiditis is 3.6 (14).

Depression doubles the risk of mortality – similar to the risk associated with smoking. Where depression is present as a comorbidity with other chronic diseases such as angina, arthritis, asthma and diabetes, it leads to a greater health-related disability than any other combination of these conditions (7).

A study by Ismail et al. that examined 253 patients with diabetes presenting to a regional centre in London with their first foot ulcer found that depression was present in 32.4% of patients, and where present it was associated with significantly higher mortality rates at 18 months (OR 2.5) (15). A strength of this study was that depression was diagnosed by formal psychiatric assessment and not just based on scores from depression scales. These findings suggest that depression may be an independent (and modifiable) risk factor for mortality in this population. Given that depression is highly treatable, its presence should be identified and targeted similar to the approach used for coexisting hypertension or hyperlipidaemia. The reality is that diabetologists are generally more confident with diagnosing and managing medical disorders than they are diagnosing and managing mental health problems including depression.

Depression: What Is It?

Depression is a mental disorder that is characterised by the following core symptoms of depressed mood, poor energy and anhedonia or loss of enjoyment. There are a number of other key features, which include biological symptoms such as sleep disturbance, change in appetite and weight and psychomotor agitation or retardation, as well as cognitive symptoms of guilt, blame, helplessness and hopelessness. In addition, there may be comorbid anxiety symptoms, comorbid psychotic symptoms or the potentially fatal symptom of suicidal ideation. Depression is categorised by severity according to the degree of symptomatology present. Severe depression may be associated with psychotic symptoms (delusions or hallucinations, characteristically congruent with mood and negative in theme). Table 2.1 shows how depressive symptoms are categorised in accordance with severity in the Tenth Revision of the International Classification of Disease and Related Health Problems (ICD-10) and the *Diagnostic and Statistical Manual of Mental Disorders*, 5th edition (DSM-5) (16, 17).

Sometimes, people with depression may also have other symptoms that are seen in other conditions. These may include various symptoms of anxiety, including generalised anxiety, panic symptoms and obsessive symptoms. In some cases of severe depression, there may be psychotic symptoms present. In depression, psychotic symptoms are usually mood-congruent, and accordingly they are negative in theme. Where delusions are present, they often are on themes such as the patient being bad or evil, severely physically ill or dying (Cotard's syndrome) or even dead, or they may include delusions of poverty or destitution. Where abnormalities of perception are present, these are often auditory hallucinations in the third or more commonly the second person. These are often derogatory in content and may have similar themes to delusions, which may or may not be present concordantly. They may tell the patient to perform certain acts, including self-harm (18).

There are many instruments that screen for depression and give a measure of depressive symptoms, but in order to make a diagnosis, a thorough diagnostic assessment is required. This includes a history of the presenting symptoms, a past psychiatric history including previous episodes of depression or elation (including treatment and treatment response), a medical history, a medication history, a family history (including of mental disorder and

Table 2.1 Categorisation of symptom severity in ICD-10 and DSM-5.

	ICD-10	DSM-5
Duration	At least 2 weeks	At least 2 weeks
Exclusion	No history of manic or hypomanic symptoms Episode not attributable to psychoactive substance use or an organic mental disorder	Symptoms do not meet criteria for a mixed episode Symptoms not due to the direct physiological effect of a substance or a general medical condition Symptoms cause clinically significant distress or functional impairment Symptoms are not better accounted for by bereavement
Symptoms	*At least 6 symptoms, including 3 core symptoms (in bold typeface):* 1 **Depressed mood** 2 **Loss of interest and enjoyment** 3 **Reduced energy** 4 Reduced energy and concentration 5 Reduced self-esteem and self-confidence 6 Ideas of guilt and unworthiness 7 Bleak and pessimistic views of the future 8 Ideas or acts of self-harm or suicide; 9 Disturbed sleep 10 Diminished appetite	*5 of 9 key symptoms:* 1 Generally depressed mood 2 Reduced pleasure or interest 3 Significant weight change (loss or gain) 4 Significant change in sleep pattern (insomnia or hypersomnia) 5 Significant change in psychomotor function (agitation or retardation) 6 Loss of energy or fatigue 7 Feelings of guilt or worthlessness 8 Reduced concentration or decisiveness 9 Recurring thoughts of death
Somatic or melancholic syndrome	*Somatic syndrome* *4 or more of the following:* Loss of interest or pleasure Lack of reactivity to pleasurable stimuli Early morning awakening (2 hours early) Objective psychomotor agitation/retardation Marked loss of appetite Weight loss (5% of body weight) Marked loss of libido	*Melancholic syndrome* Loss of pleasure Lack of reactivity to pleasurable stimuli *And 3 or more of the following:* Distinct quality of depressed mood Mood worse in morning Early morning awakening Marked psychomotor agitation or retardation Significant anorexia or weight loss Excessive or inappropriate guilt
Atypical depression	Not described	*Mood reactivity* *2 or more of the following* Significant weight gain or increase in appetite Hypersomnia Leaden paralysis Interpersonal rejection sensitivity

suicide), a personal history including life course, major events and psychological development, current social circumstances, personality (including habits) and a mental state examination. A physical examination and relevant investigations should be completed as appropriate to rule out medical differential diagnoses. An assessment for the diagnosis of depression should also assess current and past substance misuse, which may exacerbate or precipitate depressive symptoms.

The other valid way of making a diagnosis is by semi-structured diagnostic interview; this is mainly used in research studies. Tools that can be used to identify symptoms of depression include Structured Clinical Interview for DSM-5 (SCID) and Structured Clinical Assessment in Neuropsychiatry (SCAN), based on DSM-5 and ICD-10. Optimal use of these tools requires the user to have undergone significant training, hence their use is limited mainly to research settings.

Diabetes and Depression

In diabetes, good self-management skills are key to achieving optimal glycaemic control and avoiding the development of complications. Outcomes may be regarded as dependent to a significant degree on the individual patient's ability to acquire and maintain good self-management skills. Psychological factors, and in particular mood, are of particular importance given the degree to which mood influences motivation, self-efficacy and self-care.

A systematic review published in 2001 found that patients with both type 1 and type 2 diabetes have an increased incidence of depression of approximately twice that of the general population (9% compared with 5%), and a still larger proportion (up to a quarter) have subclinical depressive symptoms (19). The authors reported that the prevalence of depression was higher in women and in clinical rather than community samples (19).

There is evidence that the relationship between diabetes and depression may be bidirectional: patients with diabetes have an increased incidence of depression and patients with depression are at increased risk of developing diabetes (11, 12, 19). In the literature, the rates reported often vary considerably due to the conflation of depressive symptoms with depressive episodes, and in some cases there is incomplete differentiation from diabetes distress, with which there is some symptomatic overlap (see further discussion in Chapter 7). This may be at least partly explained by the psychological burden of living with a chronic condition (20).

Similarly, a meta-analysis that examined the effect of depression on the future development of diabetes in 2.5 million pooled participants reported that patients with depression are at a 41% higher risk of developing prediabetes and type 2 diabetes, with regional variations noted, probably due to methodological factors in the constituent studies (21).

People with diabetes and depression are more likely to have poorer outcomes, with poorer glycaemic control, greater rates of diabetic complications and higher mortality rates. This suggests that depression may be regarded as a modifiable risk factor for the morbidity and mortality in diabetes due to its role as a barrier to optimal self-management (15).

These poor outcomes may be related to difficulties with interest, motivation and energy, all of which are associated with depression and pose difficulties for optimal diabetes self-management. In particular, lifestyle modification, which is an important part of the management of diabetes, can be difficult to accomplish in patients with comorbid depression. Dysregulation of the hypothalamic–pituitary–adrenal axis has been proposed as a common pathway for both and is discussed in more detail in Chapter 5. In recent years, a common inflammatory pathway for both conditions has been discussed. While type 1 diabetes is an autoimmune condition, type 2 diabetes has been associated with acute-phase inflammatory response (22). Inflammatory response has likewise been associated with depression, with increased levels of pro-inflammatory cytokines including IL-1, IL-6, TNF, CRP and MCP-1 (23). There is preliminary evidence to suggest that this relationship may be stronger in women with type 2 diabetes (24).

Is diabetes distress associated with depression in diabetes? Certainly people with depression are likely to report poorer quality of life and higher rates of diabetes-associated distress, although no studies have established a direction to this relationship or ascertained whether depression may increase the risk of diabetes distress or vice versa. We discuss diabetes distress more comprehensively in Chapter 7.

Thyroid Disorders and Depression

Low mood is a common symptom of hypothyroidism, and where low mood and fatigue are due to thyroid dysfunction these symptoms usually resolve with treatment of the underlying cause, without the need for any depression-specific treatments. Likewise in hyperthyroidism, the presentation may mimic generalised anxiety disorder or even an agitated depression (i.e. a subtype of depression characterised by increased rather than reduced psychomotor activity). Siegmann et al. found that autoimmune thyroiditis was associated with depression and anxiety with ORs of 3.6 and 2.3, respectively (14). Identification and treatment of thyroid dysfunction is an important part of the investigation of depression, especially in elderly patients. However, thyroid dysfunction and depression may coexist, and following treatment mood and anxiety should be monitored. Thyroid disorders and their relationship with mental health are further discussed in Chapter 6.

Diagnosing Depression

Diagnostic Challenges and Overshadowing

Common depressive symptoms such as insomnia, anorexia and fatigue are also common to medical conditions, such as hyperglycaemia in diabetes. Diagnosis of depression, where there are medical comorbidities, is more complex, and clinical judgement is required to decide on the attribution of these symptoms. While on the one hand it is necessary to exclude medical causes of depressed mood, the diagnosis of depression in patients with comorbid medical conditions may be complicated by the presence of symptoms that may be common to the physical condition in question and to depression. For example, a person with diabetes may present with changes in appetite, nocturia and fatigue due to hyperglycaemia.

The other important aspect of diagnostic overshadowing is where, in an individual with an established history of a psychiatric condition such as depression, all physical symptoms are attributed to the depressive illness, rather than being considered as symptoms worthy of investigation in their own right. This may be related to cognitive biases on the part of the clinician, but perhaps may also include other factors relating to the doctor–patient communication. Differing patterns of care between people with and without mental illness have been identified that are not dissimilar to those in other marginalised groups. If this is related to bias, it is a dangerous bias, as it may contribute to the significant differential in life expectancy between people with and without mental illnesses (25).

In order to ensure that on the one hand comorbid depression is being appropriately identified and treated and conversely that every symptom that may have another aetiology is not being inappropriately attributed to depression, it is key to step back and look at the bigger picture. In particular, if cognitive or emotional symptoms of depression are present, such as inappropriate guilt or hopelessness, the possibility of depression contributing to other physical symptoms needs to be considered. Where suicidal ideation is present, this should be carefully evaluated.

Role of Screening

Screening is not merely an exercise in identifying a condition; screening involves earlier diagnosis in combination with earlier treatment and (presumed) better and more cost-effective outcomes. The use of screening for depression is controversial. A Cochrane review of screening for depression in the general population found no benefit associated with the practice of screening and no improvements in rates of treatment of depression when there are no treatment pathways implemented alongside the screening programme (26). Petrak et al. similarly concluded that when there are no tailored treatment pathways available for those people who screen positive, it is difficult to justify this practice from either an ethical or a financial perspective (27). Some clinicians may perceive screening to be inconsistent with patient-centred care (28).

Any screening process needs to consider the benefit of identifying cases that might otherwise not be detected. It also needs to avoid being onerous – being burdensome to patients or the clinicians working in the setting where it is being used. In 2006, Gilbody and colleagues found that the relative merits of screening for mental health problems are frequently overstated and that there is little convincing evidence that screening improves outcomes (29). They attribute this to a number of contributing factors, such as the undetected 'depression' often being a fluctuating or fleeting distress due to life events rather than a depressive illness (overdiagnosis). Any psychological difficulties (including depressive episodes) that are detected by this means are likely to be mild, and interventions that have a strong evidence base for a depressive disorder (structured psychotherapies and antidepressant medications) may not be effective in this population (30). Indeed, much subclinical distress is self-limiting. Gilbody and Beck discuss the differences between different screening methods, concluding that while 'stand-alone' screening is of limited benefit, screening embedded within enhanced care results in significant improvements in depression outcomes (31). In other words, where there is a system of communicating the results and providing evidence-based treatments as part of an integrated care pathway, patients have better outcomes.

There is insufficient evidence to support the routine use of screening for depression in medical outpatient clinics. However, physicians with a better conceptual understanding of mental illness make more accurate diagnoses, as do those who demonstrate empathy, who ask about family and social problems and who encourage a patient to talk with broad, open questions related to emotional issues such as coping.

It is useful to consider depression where there is evidence of difficulty coping or multiple unexplained symptoms, chronic pain or evidence of poor concordance with management of their primary condition. In particular, it is useful to have a high index of suspicion for depression where there is evidence of impairment of functioning. It may be useful to use a structured questionnaire as an aide-memoire. On the whole, improving access to treatments for depression where present and providing integrated or collaborative care are, on balance, likely to be better uses of scarce resources than simply providing a screening programme.

However, given the prevalence of depression in diabetes and its impact on outcomes including complications, should diabetologists be screening for depression? The evidence would suggest that in the absence of a pathway for diagnostic assessment and treatment this is likely to be of benefit. However, patients will benefit from treatment in terms of both their mental health and well-being and their physical health if we regard depression as a modifiable risk factor for complications. Having a high index of suspicion for depression in patients with diabetes is likely to be quite subjective and to vary between clinicians. There may be considerable benefit to having a well-organised screening system where there is a clear plan for further management if symptoms of depression or anxiety are identified.

Management of Depression in Chronic Illness

Most guidelines agree on the key treatments for uncomplicated depression (i.e. medications and psychotherapy). Medications include selective serotonin reuptake inhibitors (SSRIs) as the primary first-line treatments, with alternatives such as serotonin and noradrenaline reuptake inhibitors (SNRIs), noradenergic and specific serotonin antidepressants (NaSSAs) and, more rarely, tricyclic antidepressants (TCAs) and monoamine oxidase inhibitors (MAOIs). The psychotherapies with the strongest evidence base are cognitive behavioural therapy (CBT) and interpersonal psychotherapy (IPT).

Before considering treatment, it is important to confirm the diagnosis and exclude any conditions where there may be diagnostic overlap. Disturbance in sleep, appetite, energy and libido are depressive symptoms, but are also common to many medical conditions. Appropriate investigation and clinical judgement are required to clarify the attribution of these symptoms.

In *Depression in Adults with a Chronic Physical Health Problem: Recognition and Management (Clinical Guideline 91)*, the National Institute for Health and Care Excellence (NICE) suggests a stepped care model with four tiers, as summarised in Figure 2.1 (32). At each tier, the interventions are tailored to not only the severity but also the chronicity of the depressive episode and whether it coexists with a medical condition.

> Depression is approximately two to three times more common in patients with a chronic physical health problem (such as cancer, heart disease or diabetes) than in people who have good physical health. A chronic physical health problem can both cause and exacerbate depression and treating depression in these patients has the potential to increase their quality of life and life expectancy. The presence of a physical illness can complicate the recognition and assessment of depression, because some symptoms are common to both mental and physical disorder. Symptoms below the threshold for a diagnosis of depression can be distressing and disabling, especially in patients with a physical health problem.
>
> Source: NICE, *Clinical Guideline 91* (32)

This final sentence is where the guidance differs from the management of depression without physical health comorbidities, and we may consider treatment of subthreshold symptoms where there is evidence of impact on self-management.

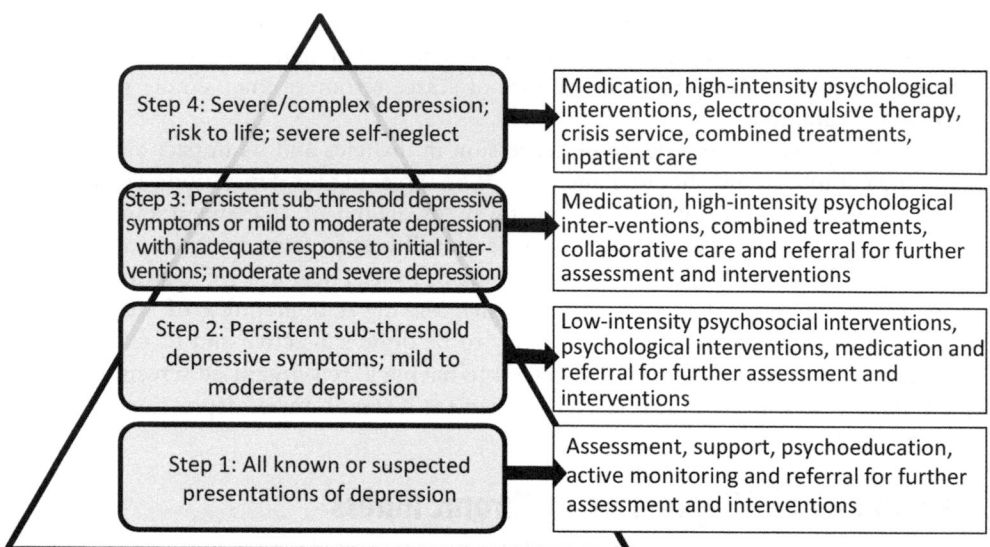

Figure 2.1 Stepped care for the management of depression with a comorbid long-term condition. Adapted from NICE, *Clinical Guideline 91* (32)

Antidepressants

In a Cochrane review, the role of antidepressants in the management of depression in people with medical conditions was examined (33). Rayner et al. stated that 'Antidepressants are effective in the treatment of depression in physically healthy populations, but there is less clarity regarding their use in physically ill patients' (33). They concluded by stating: 'This review provides evidence that antidepressants are superior to placebo in treating depression in physical illness. However, it is likely that publication and reporting biases exaggerated the effect sizes obtained. Further research is required to determine the comparative efficacy and acceptability of particular antidepressants in this population.'

Prescribing Antidepressants

In managing comorbid depression with diabetes or other chronic illness, general prescribing principles apply. Sertraline (an SSRI) and mirtazapine (a NaSSA) are usually considered first-line agents because of their favourable side-effect profiles, although it is important to bear in mind that mirtazapine may cause weight gain, which may not be ideal in all patients. Regardless of the medication chosen, it is important to ensure that a therapeutic dose is prescribed and an adequate trial given at a therapeutic dose. In choosing an antidepressant, it is important to consider the potential impact of treatment on physical health conditions and the potential for interactions with other medications.

A number of antidepressants, including duloxetine, amitriptyline and nortriptyline, are licensed for the treatment of neuropathic pain. These may be considered for patients who have comorbid depression and neuropathic pain. Pregabalin is also licensed for the treatment of neuropathic pain and may be indicated for comorbid neuropathy and anxiety.

Patients may feel some increase in anxiety or agitation in the first two weeks of SSRI treatment, despite these medications being indicated and licenced for the management of anxiety disorders. It is important that patients are advised of this and told that it will likely be transient. Prompt follow-up is important to ensure that any transient side effects are appropriately managed, with guidelines recommending review within two weeks, or one week if aged under 30 years or at risk of suicide. If you are in secondary care and unable to arrange this in your clinic system, it may be possible to ask the patient to attend their primary care doctor within two weeks and include this in the clinic letter (34).

The evidence for an association between antidepressants and glucose regulation is unclear, with case reports of both increased and decreased glucose associated with various antidepressant agents (35). Derijks et al. reported a 1.5-fold increase in the risk of hyperglycaemia and a 1.8-fold increase in the risk of hypoglycaemia associated with antidepressant medications (36). The same authors showed that long-term antidepressant use (>3 years) in diabetes was associated with a 2.8-fold increase in the risk for severe hypoglycaemia in a case–control study (36). This study found that hypoglycaemia was associated with antidepressants with high affinity for serotonin reuptake transporters (i.e. SSRIs and clomipramine). Hyperglycaemia was more strongly associated with anti-depressants that have affinity for the 5-HT$_{2c}$ (serotonin) receptor, the H$_1$ (histamine) receptor and the noradrenaline reuptake transporters (i.e. medications that include ami-triptyline, doxepin, imipramine, maprotiline, nortriptyline, mianserin and mirtazapine) (36, 37). There is evidence that fluoxetine (an SSRI) may augment cellular glucose uptake and increase cerebral glucose transporter activity in *in vitro* models, but this is yet to be confirmed in clinical populations (38). Initial studies suggested that there may be a mechanism whereby antidepressants might act directly on reducing insulin resistance, but this has not been replicated in subsequent studies in people with diabetes (39, 40).

In prescribing an antidepressant, it is important to consider other common side effects. Prescribers should consider the risk of QTc prolongation and perform an electrocardio-gram if the patient is at high risk of this. If the patient is concurrently prescribed an non-steroidal anti-inflammatory drug (NSAID) or is at high risk of gastrointestinal bleeding, use SSRIs with caution and consider gastroprotection if their use is unavoidable (41).

Psychological Therapies

NICE guidelines recommend that evidence-based psychological treatments are offered at all levels of treatment for depression. CBT has a strong evidence base and, in addition to being accessed as part of secondary care mental health services, it is now increasingly available in primary care. In the UK, the Improving Access to Psychological Therapies (IAPT) pro-gramme provides various levels of CBT and CBT-based self-help at a primary care level, available to all, free at the point of access. There is a long-term conditions pathway in the IAPT programme that may be suitable for patients who require psychological therapy. At higher levels of complexity, the patient may require input from a clinical psychologist or health psychologist or multidisciplinary treatment from a liaison psychiatry team or psychological medicine service.

Collaborative Care

There is evolving evidence of the value of integrated or collaborative care – the evidence base for this has developed mainly in the area of comorbid depression and diabetes. Katon et al. developed the TEAMcare model in Seattle, which integrated the guideline-based management of depression with the management of diabetes and/or coronary heart disease

(42). In a randomised controlled trial (RCT) comparing this intervention to usual care, Katon et al. found significant improvements in glycated haemoglobin, lipids, depression scores and cost-effectiveness (42). Another (non-randomised) integrated care model in London found significant improvements in HbA1c, but without the improved cost efficiencies hoped for (43). A systematic review by Atlantis et al. found seven RCTs and concluded that collaborative or integrated care significantly improved depression and glycaemic control in individuals with diabetes and depression (44). However, the overall weighted mean difference was small, and the authors noted that most of these studies were conducted in the USA and may not be generalisable to other healthcare settings. Coventry et al. reported on a clustered (by general practice) randomised trial in the UK. This research found a modest improvement in depressive symptoms at four months, but it did not examine glycaemic control or physical health outcomes, and it excluded patients with severe mental disorders (45). Collaborative care seems to be an intuitive way of delivering the more complex care suggested at the tip of the NICE pyramid (see Figure 2.1).

Conclusion

Depression is a common mental illness and a leading cause of burden of disease worldwide as measured by disease-adjusted life-years. When comorbid with physical illness, depression has a significant effect on recovery and even mortality. It is also more common in people with chronic physical disorders including endocrine conditions, especially diabetes, where it may be regarded as a risk factor for poorer outcomes. Comorbid mental disorders with endocrine conditions may present challenges both for the patient and for their healthcare providers, and it is important that these are identified and treated. There is some evidence for the effectiveness of joint interventions and for integrating mental and physical healthcare in collaborative models.

References

1 WHO. *Global Burden of Disease*. World Health Organization, 2004.

2 Berkman LF, Blumenthal J, Burg M, Carney RM, Catellier D, Cowan MJ, et al. Effects of treating depression and low perceived social support on clinical events after myocardial infarction: the Enhancing Recovery in Coronary Heart Disease Patients (ENRICHD) randomized trial. *JAMA*. 2003; 289(23): 3106–16.

3 Joynt KE, O'Connor CM. Lessons from SADHART, ENRICHD, and other trials. *Psychosom Med*. 2005; 67(Suppl. 1): S63–6.

4 WHO. *The Global Burden of Disease: 2004 Update*. World Health Organization, 2004.

5 Kessler RC, Bromet EJ. The epidemiology of depression across cultures. *Annu Rev Public Health*. 2013; 34: 119–38.

6 Cuijpers P, Smit F. Excess mortality in depression: a meta-analysis of community studies. *J Affect Disord*. 2002; 72(3): 227–36.

7 Moussavi S, Chatterji S, Verdes E, Tandon A, Patel V, Ustun B. Depression, chronic diseases, and decrements in health: results from the World Health Surveys. *Lancet*. 2007; 370(9590): 851–8.

8 Eaton WW, Anthony JC, Gallo J, Cai G, Tien A, Romanoski A, et al. Natural history of Diagnostic Interview Schedule/DSM-IV major depression. The Baltimore Epidemiologic Catchment Area follow-up. *Arch Gen Psychiatry*. 1997; 54 (11): 993–9.

9 Kessler RC, Chiu WT, Demler O. Prevalence, severity, and comorbidity of 12-month DSM-IV disorders in the National Comorbidity Survey Replication. *Arch Gen Psychiatry*. 2005; 62: 617–27.

10 Kendler KS, Neale MC, Kessler RC, Heath AC, Eaves LJ. The lifetime history of major depression in women. Reliability of diagnosis and heritability. *Arch Gen Psychiatry*. 1993; 50(11): 863–70.

11 Barnard KD, Skinner TC, Peveler R. The prevalence of co-morbid depression in adults with type 1 diabetes: systematic literature review. *Diabet Med*. 2006; 23(4): 445–8.

12 Ali S, Stone MA, Peters JL, Davies MJ, Khunti K. The prevalence of co-morbid depression in adults with type 2 diabetes: a systematic review and meta-analysis. *Diabet Med*. 2006; 23(11): 1165–73.

13 Weber T, Eberle J, Messelhauser U, Schiffmann L, Nies C, Schabram J, et al. Parathyroidectomy, elevated depression scores, and suicidal ideation in patients with primary hyperparathyroidism: results of a prospective multicenter study. *JAMA Surg*. 2013; 148(2): 109–15.

14 Siegmann EM, Muller HHO, Luecke C, Philipsen A, Kornhuber J, Gromer TW. Association of depression and anxiety disorders with autoimmune thyroiditis: a systematic review and meta-analysis. *JAMA Psychiatry*. 2018; 75(6): 577–84.

15 Ismail K, Winkley K, Stahl D, Chalder T, Edmonds M. A cohort study of people with diabetes and their first foot ulcer: the role of depression on mortality. *Diabetes Care*. 2007; 30(6): 1473–9.

16 APA. *The Diagnostic and Statistical Manual of Mental Disorders (5th ed – DSM-5)*. American Psychiatric Publishing, 2013.

17 WHO. *The ICD-10 Classification of Mental and Behavioural Disorders: Clinical Descriptions and Diagnostic Guidelines*. World Health Organization, 1992.

18 Casey P, Kelly B. *Fish's Clinical Psychopathology: Signs and Symptoms in Psychiatry*. RCPsych Publications, 2007.

19 Anderson RJ, Freedland KE, Clouse RE, Lustman PJ. The prevalence of comorbid depression in adults with diabetes: a meta-analysis. *Diabetes Care*. 2001; 24(6): 1069–78.

20 Penckofer S, Ferrans CE, Velsor-Friedrich B, Savoy S. The psychological impact of living with diabetes: women's day-to-day experiences. *Diabetes Educ*. 2007; 33(4): 680–90.

21 Yu M, Zhang X, Lu F, Fang L. Depression and risk for diabetes: a meta-analysis. *Can J Diabetes*. 2015; 39(4): 266–72.

22 Wang X, Bao W, Liu J, Ouyang YY, Wang D, Rong S, et al. Inflammatory markers and risk of type 2 diabetes: a systematic review and meta-analysis. *Diabetes Care*. 2013; 36 (1): 166–75.

23 Young JJ, Bruno D, Pomara N. A review of the relationship between proinflammatory cytokines and major depressive disorder. *J Affect Disord*. 2014; 169: 15–20.

24 Moulton CD, Pickup JC, Rokakis AS, Amiel SA, Ismail K, Stahl D. The prospective association between inflammation and depressive symptoms in type 2 diabetes stratified by sex. *Diabetes Care*. 2019; 42(10): 1865–72.

25 Jones S, Howard L, Thornicroft G. 'Diagnostic overshadowing': worse physical health care for people with mental illness. *Acta Psychiatr Scand*. 2008; 118(3): 169–71.

26 Gilbody S, House AO, Sheldon TA. Screening and case finding instruments for depression. *Cochrane Database Syst Rev*. 2005; (4): CD002792.

27 Petrak F, Röhrig B, Ismail K. Depression and diabetes. In: *Endotext [Internet]* (eds. KR Feingold, B Anawalt, A Boyce, G Chrousos, WW de Herder, K Dungan, et al., eds.). MDText.com, Inc., 2018. Available from: www.ncbi.nlm.nih.gov/books/NBK498652.

28 Alderson SL, Russell AM, McLintock K, Potrata B, House A, Foy R. Incentivised case finding for depression in patients with chronic heart disease and diabetes in primary care: an ethnographic study. *BMJ Open*. 2014; 4(8): e005146.

29 Gilbody S, Sheldon T, Wessely S. Should we screen for depression? *BMJ*. 2006; 332 (7548): 1027–30.

30 Gilbody SM, House AO, Sheldon TA. Routinely administered questionnaires for

depression and anxiety: systematic review. *BMJ*. 2001; 322(7283): 406–9.

31 Gilbody S, Beck D. Implementing screening as part of enhanced care: screening alone is not enough. In: *Screening for Depression in Clinical Practice: An Evidence-based Guide* (eds. AJ Mitchell, JC Coyne). Oxford University Press, 2010, pp. 123–42.

32 NICE. *Depression in Adults with a Chronic Physical Health Problem: Recognition and Management (Clinical Guideline 91)*. National Institute for Health and Care Excellence, 2009.

33 Rayner L, Price A, Evans A, Valsraj K, Higginson IJ, Hotopf M. Antidepressants for depression in physically ill people. *Cochrane Database Syst Rev*. 2010; (3): CD007503.

34 NICE. *Depression: The Treatment and Management of Depression in Adults (Clinical Guideline 90)*. National Institute for Health and Care Excellence, 2009.

35 Khoza S, Barner JC. Glucose dysregulation associated with antidepressant agents: an analysis of 17 published case reports. *Int J Clin Pharm*. 2011; 33(3): 484–92.

36 Derijks HJ, Heerdink ER, De Koning FH, Janknegt R, Klungel OH, Egberts AC. The association between antidepressant use and hypoglycaemia in diabetic patients: a nested case-control study. *Pharmacoepidemiol Drug Saf*. 2008; 17(4): 336–44.

37 Derijks HJ, Meyboom RH, Heerdink ER, De Koning FH, Janknegt R, Lindquist M, et al. The association between antidepressant use and disturbances in glucose homeostasis: evidence from spontaneous reports. *Eur J Clin Pharmacol*. 2008; 64(5): 531–8.

38 Stapel B, Gorinski N, Gmahl N, Rhein M, Preuss V, Hilfiker-Kleiner D, et al. Fluoxetine induces glucose uptake and modifies glucose transporter palmitoylation in human peripheral blood mononuclear cells. *Expert Opin Ther Targets*. 2019; 23(10): 883–91.

39 Weber-Hamann B, Gilles M, Lederbogen F, Heuser I, Deuschle M. Improved insulin sensitivity in 80 nondiabetic patients with MDD after clinical remission in a double-blind, randomized trial of amitriptyline and paroxetine. *J Clin Psychiatry*. 2006; 67(12): 1856–61.

40 Pyykkonen AJ, Raikkonen K, Tuomi T, Eriksson JG, Groop L, Isomaa B. Depressive symptoms, antidepressant medication use, and insulin resistance: the PPP-Botnia study. *Diabetes Care*. 2011; 34(12): 2545–7.

41 Dalton SO, Sorensen HT, Johansen C. SSRIs and upper gastrointestinal bleeding: what is known and how should it influence prescribing? *CNS Drugs*. 2006; 20(2): 143–51.

42 Katon WJ, Lin EH, Von Korff M, Ciechanowski P, Ludman EJ, Young B, et al. Collaborative care for patients with depression and chronic illnesses. *N Engl J Med*. 2010; 363(27): 2611–20.

43 Ismail K, Stewart K, Ridge K, Britneff E, Freudenthal R, Stahl D, et al. A pilot study of an integrated mental health, social and medical model for diabetes care in an inner-city setting: Three Dimensions for Diabetes (3DFD). *Diabet Med*. 2020; 37(10): 1658–68.

44 Atlantis E, Fahey P, Foster J. Collaborative care for comorbid depression and diabetes: a systematic review and meta-analysis. *BMJ Open*. 2014; 4(4): e004706.

45 Coventry P, Lovell K, Dickens C, Bower P, Chew-Graham C, McElvenny D, et al. Integrated primary care for patients with mental and physical multimorbidity: cluster randomised controlled trial of collaborative care for patients with depression comorbid with diabetes or cardiovascular disease. *BMJ*. 2015; 350: h638.

Antipsychotic Medications and Metabolic Syndrome

Aoife M. Egan and Anne M. Doherty

Metabolic Syndrome: Diagnosis and Clinical Implications

The term 'metabolic syndrome' is used to describe a cluster of risk factors for type 2 diabetes and cardiovascular disease. Other names commonly used for the same entity include 'syndrome X' and 'insulin resistance syndrome'. Although many definitions exist, a number of organisations, including the American Heart Association and the International Association for the Study of Obesity, have proposed criteria for diagnosing metabolic syndrome based on waist circumference, blood pressure and measures of fasting glucose, triglycerides and high-density lipoprotein (HDL) cholesterol (1). These criteria are further detailed in Table 3.1.

The syndrome is becoming increasingly common, particularly in light of the current obesity pandemic, as elevated weight is a major risk factor. In the USA, for example, data from the National Health and Nutrition Examination Survey (NHANES) reports that 34.5% of participants met the criteria for metabolic syndrome in the 1999–2002 survey compared to 22.0% in the 1988–94 survey (2, 3).

There is a strong association between the presence of metabolic syndrome and the risk of developing type 2 diabetes. A 2008 meta-analysis of multiple, diverse cohorts reported relative risks ranging from 3.53 to 5.17 (4). Likewise, for cardiovascular disease, metabolic syndrome is reported to increase the relative risk of cardiovascular events and death by a factor of 1.78 (5). Identifying a patient as having metabolic syndrome allows for intervention to reduce the development of type 2 diabetes and/or cardiovascular disease. This typically takes the form of aggressive lifestyle changes with or without pharmacological intervention to target specific components of the syndrome.

It is worth noting that there has actually been significant criticism of the use of the term 'metabolic syndrome'. This centres around the limited evidence for setting its definitions and the fact that the associated cardiovascular risk has not been shown to be greater than the sum of its individual components (6–8). Despite this, the description continues to be used frequently by healthcare professionals worldwide, and metabolic syndrome does appear to be highly prevalent among individuals with severe mental illness.

Association of Metabolic Syndrome with Severe Mental Illness

Patients with severe mental illness are at increased risk for metabolic syndrome, diabetes and cardiovascular disease. This is likely due to a number of factors, including higher rates of smoking, poor diet and disordered lifestyle with minimal physical activity (9). In addition, this population is less likely to receive prompt diagnosis and treatment for modifiable risk factors such as hypertension, dyslipidaemia and prediabetes (10). As outlined in Chapter 10, there appears to be a bidirectional relationship between obesity

Table 3.1 Criteria for the diagnosis of metabolic syndrome.

Any 3 of the following 5 criteria:
(1) Elevated waist circumference using population- and country-specific definitions
(2) Fasting glucose $\geq$5.5mmol/L (100 mg/dL) or Rx
(3) Triglycerides $\geq$1.7mmol/L (150 mg/dL) or Rx
(4) HDL cholesterol: <1.0 mmol/L (40 mg/dL) (male), <1.3 mmol/L (50 mg/dL) (female) or Rx
(5) $\geq$130 mmHg systolic or $\geq$85 mmHg diastolic or Rx
HDL: high-density lipoprotein; Rx: pharmacological treatment.

and mood disorders, and patients with schizophrenia are also at significant risk of obesity. Interestingly, patients with schizophrenia were observed to have an elevated risk of type 2 diabetes, even before antipsychotic medications became the mainstay of therapy (9, 11). There are a number of chromosomal regions common to both type 2 diabetes and schizophrenia, suggesting the potential for a genetic link (12).

It is clear, however, that the pharmacological approach to the treatment of severe mental illness also contributes to the development of metabolic syndrome in this susceptible group of individuals. Although the primary indication for antipsychotic medications is schizophrenia and related disorders, these drugs are also used in the context of severe mood disorders such as bipolar and unipolar depression (13). These medications can be broadly classified into first- and second-generation agents. Overall, first- and second-generation agents appear to be similar with regards to efficacy, but the second-generation agents induce fewer extrapyramidal side effects (14). Compared to the first-generation medications, atypical (or second-generation) agents have a lower affinity for dopamine D_2 receptors and greater affinities for alternative neuroreceptors, including those for serotonin and norepinephrine. As outlined in Table 3.2, antipsychotic medications are heterogeneous in terms of their effects on metabolic risk, but many have a propensity to induce weight gain and are associated with significant effects on lipid and/or glucose metabolism abnormalities in adults (13).

Antipsychotic Medications and Weight Gain

Weight gain is a well-described side effect of antipsychotic medications and can contribute to the development of each of the individual metabolic syndrome components. Among the first-generation agents, chlorpromazine and thioridazine are associated with the greatest risk of weight gain; however, this effect tends to be more prominent among the second-generation agents – with the exception of aripiprazole and zisprasidone (14). In particular, clozapine and olanzapine are associated with a substantial risk of weight gain (Table 3.2). The greater effect of second-generation agents on weight gain appears to stem from their blockade of hypothalamic histamine 1 (H_1) and serotonin 2C (5-HT_{2c}) receptors, which leads to increased appetite (9).

Clinical predictors of antipsychotic-related weight gain include a family history of obesity, personal factors including younger age and non-white ethnicity and treatment-related factors including higher drug dose and polypharmacy (13). The greatest risk period for weight gain seems to be in the first few months of treatment in a drug-naïve patient. For

Table 3.2 Metabolic risks associated with antipsychotic drugs.

Antipsychotic drug	Potency	Associated risk of weight gain	Associated risk of lipid and/or glucose metabolism abnormalities
First-generation agents			
Chorpromazine	Low	Substantial	High (limited data)
Fluphenazine	High	Neutral/low	Low (limited data)
Haloperidol	High	Neutral/low	Low
Molindone	Mid	Neutral	Low (limited data)
Perphenazine	Mid	Neutral/low	Low
Pimozide	High	Neutral/low	Low (limited data)
Thioridazine	Low	Intermediate	High (limited data)
Second-generation agents			
Amisulpride	NA	Neutral/low	Mild
Aripiprazole	NA	Neutral/low	Low
Asenapine	NA	Low	Low (limited data)
Clozapine	NA	Substantial	High
Iloperidone	NA	Intermediate	Mild (limited data)
Lurasidone	NA	Neutral/low	Low (limited data)
Olanzapine	NA	Substantial	High
Paliperidone	NA	Intermediate	Mild
Quetiapine	NA	Intermediate	Moderate
Risperidone	NA	Intermediate	Mild
Sertindole	NA	Intermediate	Mild
Ziprasidone	NA	Neutral/low	Low
Zotepine	NA	Intermediate	NR

NA: not applicable; NR: not reported.
Adapted from De Hert et al. (13)

example, a meta-analysis reported weight gain of 3.8 kg and an increase of 1.2 body mass index (BMI) points within the first 12 weeks of treatment in antipsychotic-naïve patients (15). A number of different pharmacological agents were used in the included studies, but risperidone and olanzapine accounted for the majority. The Clinical Antipsychotic Trials of Intervention Effectiveness (CATIE) included patients with chronic schizophrenia and mean disease duration of 14 years and mean duration of follow-up of 18 months (16). The aim of the study was to determine differences in the overall effectiveness of five antipsychotic medications. Clinically significant weight gain was defined as weight gain of at least 7%, and this was highest for olanzapine (30%), followed by quetiapine (16%), risperidone (14%), perphenazine (12%) and ziprasidone (7%).

Contribution of Antipsychotic Medications to Metabolic Syndrome Components

It is difficult to determine the precise contribution of individual antipsychotic medications to features of metabolic syndrome within 'real-life' cohorts. Any observations will be associated with a number of confounding variables, including baseline patient characteristics and prescriber preferences. For example, a prescriber's choice of antipsychotic agent may be influenced by the patient's baseline BMI or cardiovascular status. One systematic review and meta-analysis of 77 publications including 25,692 subjects with schizophrenia noted an overall rate of metabolic syndrome of 32.5% (95% confidence interval (CI) = 30.1–35.0%) (17). The strongest associated risk was illness duration (adjusted R^2: 0.35, $p < 0.0001$), and the highest rates of metabolic syndrome were seen in those prescribed clozapine (52%), olanzapine (28.2%) and risperidone (27.9%), with the lowest rates seen in those who were not medicated (20%). These findings suggest that choice of individual antipsychotic drug and duration of therapy are key factors in determining whether metabolic syndrome will develop in an individual patient.

The effect of antipsychotic medications on blood pressure is not clear. A retrospective study found that olanzapine and risperidone raised blood pressure during the first three days after initiation, but clozapine reduced blood pressure (18). Prospective studies are required for further evaluation of this, but even if there is not a direct effect on blood pressure, medication-induced weight gain will contribute to an increased risk of hypertension.

On the other hand, antipsychotic-associated dyslipidaemia can occur independently of weight gain. Chlorpromazine and other phenothiazines appear to preferentially elevate triglycerides but also to elevate total cholesterol. Butyrophenone derivatives such as haloperidol appear to have a more neutral effect on serum lipids (19). This is exemplified in a study of long-term hospitalised men with schizophrenia where significant elevations in serum triglyceride concentrations were observed in those receiving phenothiazines (mean 163 ± 65 mg/dL) compared to those receiving butyrophenones (mean 104 ± 52 mg/dL) (20). Among the second-generation agents, olanzapine, clozapine and quetiapine are associated with increases in serum triglycerides and in concentrations of low-density lipoprotein and non-HDL cholesterol (13). Indeed, the development of severe hypertriglyceridaemia (>500 mg/dL) has been described in association with these three agents in the absence of dramatic weight gain (21, 22). Among the newer agents, ziprasidone, aripiprazole and risperidone appear to have a more neutral effect on lipid profiles. Mechanistically, the pathways leading to such lipid disturbances have not been fully elucidated, but it has been suggested that medication-induced alterations in peroxisome proliferator-activated receptors and progesterone receptor membrane component 1/insulin-induced gene 2 may directly lead to increased lipid biosynthesis in the liver (23–25).

As is summarised in Table 3.2, individual antipsychotic medications are associated with a variable risk of impaired glucose metabolism. Chlorpromazine, clozapine and olanzapine feature as high-risk medications in this regard. A large Danish registry study reported that compared with unexposed individuals, treatment with first-generation antipsychotics (rate ratio (RR) = 1.53, 95% CI = 1.49–1.56) as well as second-generation antipsychotics (RR = 1.32, 95% CI = 1.22–1.42) is associated with increased risk of subsequent incident diabetes (26). Although the findings must be interpreted in the setting of prescribing and reporting biases, a report from a US Food and Drug Administration (FDA) database of adverse events described adjusted reporting ratios (CIs) for diabetes mellitus for various antipsychotic agents as follows: olanzapine 9.6 (9.2–10.0), risperidone 3.8 (3.5–4.1), quetiapine 3.5 (3.2–3.9), clozapine 3.1 (2.9–3.3), ziprasidone 2.4 (2.0–2.9), aripiprazole 2.4 (1.9–2.9) and haloperidol 2.0 (1.7–2.3) (27). Interestingly, another large registry study found that the association between antipsychotic drug use and diabetes mellitus was stronger in younger patients: for patients aged 0–24 years, the odds ratio was 8.9 (95% CI = 7.0–11.3) compared to an odds ratio of 1.3 (1.2–1.4) for those aged 55–64 years (28). These findings may relate to the fact that additional biological variables (including age) become more dominant as a patient gets older and minimise the independent effect of the antipsychotic medications (13). More recently, Zhang et al. conducted a network meta-analysis to create a hierarchy of the effects of 12 antipsychotic agents on blood glucose levels. They found that only olanzapine was associated with significantly increased glucose levels compared to a placebo (mean difference = 3.95, 95% CI = 0.14–7.76) (29). Although it was initially assumed that antipsychotics increased the risk of diabetes simply by promoting weight gain, there is now significant evidence that antipsychotics directly decrease insulin sensitivity and insulin secretory capacity (30).

A key study by Ader et al. examined the effects of olanzapine and risperidone (versus placebo) on adiposity, insulin sensitivity and pancreatic beta-cell function in dogs (31). Olanzepine (but not risperidone) was found to increase both insulin resistance and adiposity (subcutaneous and visceral) and there was a failure of beta-cell compensation. This well-designed study provided crucial insights into the diabetogenic effects of the atypical antipsychotics. Subsequent *in vitro* experiments have identified potential pathways by which antipsychotics may impair insulin sensitivity, such as attenuating insulin-induced phosphorylation of insulin-like growth factor receptors in fibroblasts and reducing insulin-stimulated glucose uptake in PC12 and L6 cells (32, 33). Additional studies have demonstrated that antipsychotics increase apoptosis of insulin-producing pancreatic beta-cells, blunt glucose-stimulated insulin release by antagonising dopamine D_2 receptors and decrease beta-cell responsiveness by blocking $5-HT_{1a}$ and M_3 muscarinic receptors (30). Indeed, these effects on insulin secretion may explain reports of diabetic ketoacidosis occurring in patients initiated on antipsychotic agents but without evidence of autoimmune type 1 diabetes (34).

Assessment and Monitoring of Metabolic Risk Factors

When choosing an antipsychotic agent, prescribers must balance the potential for adverse outcomes with the likely therapeutic benefit of the medication. For certain patients, this means that an agent with a high risk of metabolic side effects cannot be avoided. In 2004, the American Diabetes Association (ADA), the American Psychiatric Association (APA), the American Association of Clinical Endocrinologists (AACE) and the North American Association for the Study of Obesity (NAASO) published a consensus statement that included recommendations on the assessment and treatment of metabolic effects in patients receiving antipsychotic medications (35). Drawing from these recommendations, the Lester Positive Cardiometabolic Health Resource endorsed by the Royal Colleges in the UK provides a helpful guide, including a graphic, which indicates the baseline and ongoing routine assessments that should be conducted and the clinical treatments to be undertaken where risks are identified (36). Key recommendations are outlined in Table 3.3.

Table 3.3 Recommended monitoring for patients on antipsychotic medications.

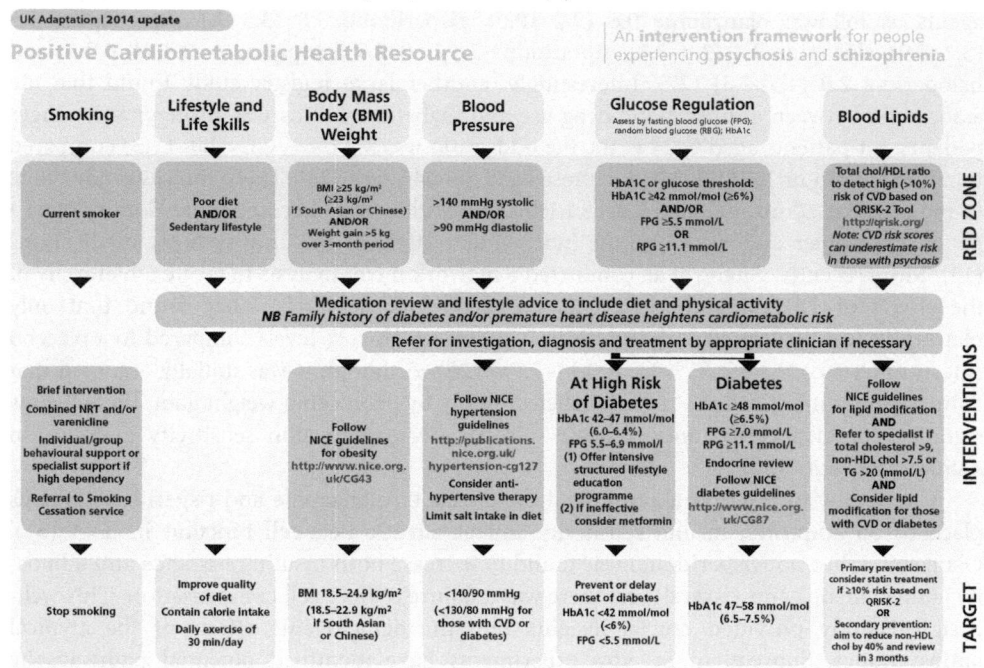

chol: cholesterol; CVD: cardiovascular disease; HDL: high-density lipoprotein; NICE: National Institute for Health and Care Excellence; NRT: nicotine replacement therapy; TG: triglycerides.
Reproduced from Shiers et al. (36). Royal College of Psychiatrists, London (with permission)

With regards to diabetes screening, HbA1c is a convenient test that is now commonly used in clinical practice to diagnose diabetes; however, it may not be significantly elevated if there is a rapid onset of hyperglycaemia, as sometimes happens after beginning antipsychotic therapy (30). In this scenario, plasma glucose is a more reliable indicator of glycaemic status. In 2009, the European Psychiatric Association (EPA), supported by the European Association for the Study of Diabetes (EASD) and the European Society of Cardiology (ESC), published a position statement on cardiovascular disease and diabetes in people with severe mental illness with a goal of increasing awareness among psychiatrists and primary care physicians caring for patients with severe mental illness to screen and treat cardiovascular risk factors (37). Similar guidance is available from local and national organisations worldwide, including the National Institute for Health and Care Excellence (NICE) in the UK (38). Unfortunately, despite these guidelines, rates of 'metabolic monitoring' at baseline remain very low in people prescribed antipsychotic medications. This is exemplified in a systematic review of 39 studies (218,940 subjects) across 5 countries that found low rates of routine baseline screening (39). Cholesterol was measured in 41.5% (95% CI = 18.0–67.3), glucose in 44.3% (95% CI = 36.3–52.4) and weight in just 47.9% (95% CI = 32.4–63.7). Slightly better adherence was noted for blood pressure, which was measured in 69.8% (95% CI = 50.9–85.8), and triglycerides, which were measured in 59.9% (95% CI = 36.6–81.1) at the time of drug initiation. Inadequacies in assessment and monitoring of risk factors result in missed opportunities for intervention and are undoubtedly contributing to the higher mortality from cardiovascular disease that is observed in patients with schizophrenia and bipolar disorder (13).

Mitigating Adverse Metabolic Effects of Antipsychotic Medications

Healthcare professionals should take every opportunity to educate their patients on the benefits of a healthy lifestyle with an emphasis on regular exercise, a balanced diet and smoking cessation if applicable (13). Nutrition and physical activity counselling should be provided for all patients who are overweight or obese (35). Prior to initiating an antipsychotic medication, patients and caregivers should be adequately informed regarding the risk of weight gain and other metabolic side effects. In those patients who have a baseline higher risk for cardiovascular complications, consideration should be given to choosing a medication with a lower propensity for adverse metabolic effects. Owing to the fact that many patients with psychotic disorders may have negative symptoms of schizophrenia, such as apathy, amotivation and reduce social drive, initiating health lifestyle changes may be particularly challenging for this patient group. Specific supports may be required (e.g. specially tailored education groups, including family and carers in education) in order to enable patients to make the lifestyle modifications required to mitigate their risk, although educational programmes may not suffice in this respect (40). On a practical level, mental health professionals are usually the health professionals who spend the greatest amount of time with patients with severe mental illness, and as such they are uniquely positioned to support patients in the lifestyle changes required (41).

Once treatment is established, a weight gain of greater than 5–7% of the baseline weight or the development of hyperglycaemia, hyperlipidaemia, hypertension or other clinically significant adverse metabolic effects should trigger medication reassessment (13, 35). A number of therapies have been assessed with regards to minimising the weight gain associated with antipsychotic agents, with most evidence being available for metformin followed by topirimate (42). These agents may be useful adjuvants in selected patients, particularly when switching the antipsychotic medication is not possible. Standard blood pressure, lipid and glycaemic targets apply equally to those with mental health disorders, and antihypertensives and lipid- and glucose-lowering medications should be introduced as required (see Chapter 13), with specialist referral where indicated. The Lester Positive Cardiometabolic Health Resource may be a useful guide in the clinical management of risk factors where identified (36).

The guidelines of the Joint British Diabetes Societies (JBDS) and Royal College of Psychiatrists suggest some practical measures at an organisational level that may help to ensure that diabetes and its risk factors are prevented or managed as well as possible. These suggestions included:

(1) Creating a diabetes register for all patients.

(2) Ensuring that a named clinical staff member is responsible for ensuring that inpatient admissions are used as an opportunity to complete as many of the screening and treatments measures as are indicated.

(3) Enhancing links between the mental health and diabetes services, such as appointing diabetes mental health nurse specialists or developing a workforce of link nurses who receive additional training in diabetes or to take on a coordinator role.

(4) Ensuring that diabetes is included in continuing professional development and training for mental health teams.
(5) Ensuring that the food provided in inpatient units meets the needs of people with diabetes. For those with obesity and type 2 diabetes not at risk of hypoglycaemia, catering staff should be encouraged to control portion sizes.
(6) Regular glucose monitoring for patients with diabetes, such as before meals or for patients who are restrained.
(7) Reviewing the rationale for the class and type of antipsychotic medication and weighing up its benefits versus its risks of obesity and diabetes in the context of each patient's diabetes risk status (41).

Additional Considerations: Hyperprolactinaemia and Antipsychotics

Both typical and, to a lesser extent, atypical antipsychotics are associated with hyperprolactinaemia. Prevalence is much higher than in the general population, where the prevalence is approximately 0.4%. In people taking antipsychotics, rates vary from 18% to 72% in men and from 42% to 93% in women (43).

Blockade of the D_2 receptors on the pituitary lactotroph cells results in the inhibition of hypothalamic dopamine, which causes hyperprolactinaemia. Hyperprolactinaemia can be asymptomatic or result in a variety of side effects, including irregular menses, infertility, male gynaecomastia, sexual dysfunction and, in the long term, osteoporosis. It was thought at one point that hyperprolactinaemia might be associated with an elevated risk of breast cancer, but more recent reviews suggest that this is less likely to be clinically significant (44). Certain antipsychotics, such as olanzapine and clozapine, are associated with a transient rise in prolactin, whereas agents such as risperidone, amisulpiride and the typical antipsychotics are associated with a more sustained elevation in serum prolactin, which relates to the rate of dissociation of the active compound from the D_2 receptors. Aripiprazole, as a partial D_2 agonist, may suppress prolactin levels in many people (45).

The guidelines are not consistent in terms of the required screening or management of hyperprolactinaemia, although in practice this is usually screened for by mental health services or in primary care, especially for high-risk groups such as adolescents, premenopausal women and people on medications that are associated with a higher risk of hyperprolactinaemia (46). Screening will ideally occur prior to treatment initiation, which will make it easier to attribute subsequent hyperprolactinaemia to drug causes (46). Where the aetiology of the hyperprolactinaemia is less clear (i.e. where there are symptoms of pituitary disease and prolactin levels >150 ng/mL, which is four times the upper limit of normal), an endocrinology opinion may be helpful. If there is low risk of mental destabilisation, the antipsychotic may be held for three to four days and a repeat level taken. A significant reduction in serum prolactin will suggest that there is unlikely to be any underlying pathology, but holding antipsychotics for this period of time may not be advisable for certain patients (47).

Where there are significant clinical manifestations of hyperprolactinaemia, it may be possible to consider adjusting the dose or switching to an alternative agent; where this is not possible, the addition of aripiprazole may effect a reduction in serum hyperprolactinaemia (48). It is important that patients are screened for osteoporosis. Replacement of testosterone in men and oestrogen in women may improve symptoms of sexual dysfunction and prevent osteoporosis. Some studies have suggested using dopamine agonists to reduce prolactin and reverse the effects of hyperprolactinaemia, but there is a risk that this may exacerbate psychotic symptoms (49).

Conclusions

Antipsychotic medications have benefitted countless people with a wide variety of psychiatric disorders. However, they do have the potential to induce metabolic disturbances in a population that is known to have a high risk of cardiovascular disease. This can result in the development of metabolic syndrome and associated complications. Overall, the second-generation antipsychotic agents have a stronger association with these adverse effects compared to their first-generation counterparts, and previously untreated patients are at the highest risk. With this in mind, healthcare professionals and patients should be well informed on this issue and institute close monitoring and prompt treatment of at-risk individuals.

References

1   Alberti KGMM, Eckel RH, Grundy SM, Zimmet PZ, Cleeman JI, Donato KA, et al. Harmonizing the metabolic syndrome: a joint interim statement of the International Diabetes Federation Task Force on Epidemiology and Prevention; National Heart, Lung, and Blood Institute; American Heart Association; World Heart Federation; International Atherosclerosis Society; and International Association for the Study of Obesity. *Circulation.* 2009; 120(16): 1640–5.

2   Ford ES, Giles WH, Dietz WH. Prevalence of the metabolic syndrome among US adults: findings from the third National Health and Nutrition Examination Survey. *JAMA.* 2002; 287(3): 356–9.

3   Ford ES. Prevalence of the metabolic syndrome defined by the International Diabetes Federation among adults in the U.S. *Diabetes Care.* 2005; 28(11): 2745–9.

4   Ford ES, Li C, Sattar N. Metabolic syndrome and incident diabetes: current state of the evidence. *Diabetes Care.* 2008; 31(9): 1898–904.

5   Gami AS, Witt BJ, Howard DE, Erwin PJ, Gami LA, Somers VK, Montori VM. Metabolic syndrome and risk of incident cardiovascular events and death: a systematic review and meta-analysis of longitudinal studies. *J Am Coll Cardiol.* 2007; 49(4): 403–14.

6   Kahn R, Buse J, Ferrannini E, Stern M, American Diabetes Association, European Association for the Study of Diabetes. The metabolic syndrome: time for a critical appraisal: joint statement from the American Diabetes Association and the European Association for the Study of Diabetes. *Diabetes Care.* 2005; 28(9): 2289–304.

7   Kahn R, Buse J, Ferrannini E, Stern M. The metabolic syndrome: time for a critical appraisal. Joint statement from the American Diabetes Association and the European Association for the Study of Diabetes. *Diabetologia.* 2005; 48(9): 1684–99.

8   Sundström J, Vallhagen E, Risérus U, Byberg L, Zethelius B, Berne C, et al. Risk associated with the metabolic syndrome versus the sum of its individual components. *Diabetes Care.* 2006; 29(7): 1673–4.

9   Pramyothin P, Khaodhiar L. Metabolic syndrome with the atypical antipsychotics. *Curr Opin Endocrinol Diabetes Obes.* 2010; 17(5): 460–6.

10 Nasrallah HA, Meyer JM, Goff DC, McEvoy JP, Davis SM, Stroup TS, Lieberman JA. Low rates of treatment for hypertension, dyslipidemia and diabetes in schizophrenia: data from the CATIE schizophrenia trial sample at baseline. *Schizophr Res.* 2006; 86(1–3): 15–22.

11 Kohen D. Diabetes mellitus and schizophrenia: historical perspective. *Br J Psychiatry Suppl.* 2004; 47: S64–6.

12 Mitchell BD. Clustering of schizophrenia with other comorbidities–what can we learn? *Schizophr Bull.* 2009; 35(2): 282–3.

13 De Hert M, Detraux J, van Winkel R, Yu W, Correll CU. Metabolic and cardiovascular adverse effects associated with antipsychotic drugs. *Nat Rev Endocrinol.* 2011; 8(2): 114–26.

14 Leucht S, Corves C, Arbter D, Engel RR, Li C, Davis JM. Second-generation versus first-generation antipsychotic drugs for schizophrenia: a meta-analysis. *Lancet.* 2009; 373(9657): 31–41.

15 Tarricone I, Gozzi BF, Serretti A, Grieco D, Berardi D. Weight gain in antipsychotic-naive patients: a review and meta-analysis. *Psychol Med.* 2010; 40(2): 187–200.

16 Lieberman JA, Stroup TS, McEvoy JP, Swartz MS, Rosenheck RA, Perkins DO, et al. Effectiveness of antipsychotic drugs in patients with chronic schizophrenia. *N Engl J Med.* 2005; 353(12): 1209–23.

17 Mitchell AJ, Vancampfort D, Sweers K, van Winkel R, Yu W, De Hert M. Prevalence of metabolic syndrome and metabolic abnormalities in schizophrenia and related disorders – a systematic review and meta-analysis. *Schizophr Bull.* 2013; 39(2): 306–18.

18 Parks KA, Parks CG, Yost JP, Bennett JI, Onwuameze OE. Acute blood pressure changes associated with antipsychotic administration to psychiatric inpatients. *Prim Care Companion CNS Disord.* 2018; 20(4): 18m02299.

19 Meyer JM, Koro CE. The effects of antipsychotic therapy on serum lipids: a comprehensive review. *Schizophr Res.* 2004; 70(1): 1–17.

20 Sasaki J, Funakoshi M, Arakawa K. Lipids and apolipoproteins in patients treated with major tranquilizers. *Clin Pharmacol Ther.* 1985; 37(6): 684–7.

21 Ghaeli P, Dufresne RL. Serum triglyceride levels in patients treated with clozapine. *Am J Health Syst Pharm.* 1996; 53(17): 2079–81.

22 Meyer JM. Novel antipsychotics and severe hyperlipidemia. *J Clin Psychopharmacol.* 2001; 21(4): 369–74.

23 Kim DD, Barr AM, Fredrikson DH, Honer WG, Procyshyn RM. Association between serum lipids and antipsychotic response in schizophrenia. *Curr Neuropharmacol.* 2019; 17(9): 852–60.

24 Cai HL, Tan QY, Jiang P, Dang RL, Xue Y, Tang MM, et al. A potential mechanism underlying atypical antipsychotics-induced lipid disturbances. *Transl Psychiatry.* 2015; 5: e661.

25 Nasrallah HA. Atypical antipsychotic-induced metabolic side effects: insights from receptor-binding profiles. *Mol Psychiatry.* 2008; 13(1): 27–35.

26 Kessing LV, Thomsen AF, Mogensen UB, Andersen PK. Treatment with antipsychotics and the risk of diabetes in clinical practice. *Br J Psychiatry.* 2010; 197 (4): 266–71.

27 Baker RA, Pikalov A, Tran Q-V, Kremenets T, Arani RB, Doraiswamy PM. Atypical antipsychotic drugs and diabetes mellitus in the US Food and Drug Administration Adverse Event database: a systematic Bayesian signal detection analysis. *Psychopharmacol Bull.* 2009; 42(1): 11–31.

28 Hammerman A, Dreiher J, Klang SH, Munitz H, Cohen AD, Goldfracht M. Antipsychotics and diabetes: an age-related association. *Ann Pharmacother.* 2008; 42 (9): 1316–22.

29 Zhang Y, Liu Y, Su Y, You Y, Ma Y, Yang G, et al. The metabolic side effects of 12 antipsychotic drugs used for the treatment of schizophrenia on glucose: a network meta-analysis. *BMC Psychiatry.* 2017; 17(1): 373.

30 Holt RIG. Association between antipsychotic medication use and diabetes. *Curr Diab Rep.* 2019; 19(10): 96.

31 Ader M, Kim SP, Catalano KJ, Ionut V, Hucking K, Richey JM, et al. Metabolic dysregulation with atypical antipsychotics occurs in the absence of underlying disease: a placebo-controlled study of olanzapine and risperidone in dogs. *Diabetes.* 2005; 54 (3): 862–71.

32 Panariello F, Perruolo G, Cassese A, Giacco F, Botta G, Barbagallo APM, et al. Clozapine impairs insulin action by up-

regulating Akt phosphorylation and Ped/Pea-15 protein abundance. *J Cell Physiol.* 2012; 227(4): 1485–92.

33   Alghamdi F, Guo M, Abdulkhalek S, Crawford N, Amith SR, Szewczuk MR. A novel insulin receptor-signaling platform and its link to insulin resistance and type 2 diabetes. *Cell Signal.* 2014; 26(6): 1355–68.

34   Polcwiartek C, Vang T, Bruhn CH, Hashemi N, Rosenzweig M, Nielsen J. Diabetic ketoacidosis in patients exposed to antipsychotics: a systematic literature review and analysis of Danish adverse drug event reports. *Psychopharmacology (Berl).* 2016; 233(21–22): 3663–72.

35   American Diabetes Association, American Psychiatric Association, American Association of Clinical Endocrinologists, North American Association for the Study of Obesity. Consensus development conference on antipsychotic drugs and obesity and diabetes. *Diabetes Care.* 2004; 27(2): 596–601.

36   Shiers D, Rafi I, Cooper SJ, Holt R. Positive Cardiometabolic Health Resource: an intervention framework for patients with psychosis and schizophrenia. 2014 update (with acknowledgement to the late Helen Lester for her contribution to the original 2012 version), 2014. Available from: www.rcpsych.ac.uk/docs/default-source/improving-care/ccqi/national-clinical-audits/ncap-library/ncap-e-version-nice-endorsed-lester-uk-adaptation.pdf?sfvrsn=39bab4_2

37   De Hert M, Dekker JM, Wood D, Kahl KG, Holt RIG, Möller H-J. Cardiovascular disease and diabetes in people with severe mental illness position statement from the European Psychiatric Association (EPA), supported by the European Association for the Study of Diabetes (EASD) and the European Society of Cardiology (ESC). *Eur Psychiatry.* 2009; 24(6): 412–24.

38   National Institute for Health and Care Excellence. Psychosis and schizophrenia in adults: prevention and management, 2014. Available from: www.nice.org.uk/guidance/cg178/chapter/1-recommendations

39   Mitchell AJ, Delaffon V, Vancampfort D, Correll CU, De Hert M. Guideline concordant monitoring of metabolic risk in people treated with antipsychotic medication: systematic review and meta-analysis of screening practices. *Psychol Med.* 2012; 42(1): 125–47.

40   Holt RI, Hind D, Gossage-Worrall R, Bradburn MJ, Saxon D, McCrone P, et al. Structured lifestyle education to support weight loss for people with schizophrenia, schizoaffective disorder and first episode psychosis: the STEPWISE RCT. *Health Technol Assess.* 2018; 22(65): 1–160.

41   Joint British Diabetes Societies for Inpatient Care and Royal College of Psychiatrists. The management of diabetes in adults and children with psychiatric disorders in inpatient settings, 2017. Available from: www.diabetes.org.uk/resources-s3/2017-10/Management of diabetes in adults and children with psychiatric disorders in inpatient settings-August-2017.pdf

42   Dayabandara M, Hanwella R, Ratnatunga S, Seneviratne S, Suraweera C, de Silva VA. Antipsychotic-associated weight gain: management strategies and impact on treatment adherence. *Neuropsychiatr Dis Treat.* 2017; 13: 2231–41.

43   Bushe C, Shaw M, Peveler RC. A review of the association between antipsychotic use and hyperprolactinaemia. *J Psychopharmacol.* 2008; 22(2 Suppl.): 46–55.

44   De Hert M, Peuskens J, Sabbe T, Mitchell AJ, Stubbs B, Neven P, et al. Relationship between prolactin, breast cancer risk, and antipsychotics in patients with schizophrenia: a critical review. *Acta Psychiatr Scand.* 2016; 133(1): 5–22.

45   Kane JM, Meltzer HY, Carson JrWH, McQuade RD, Marcus RN, Sanchez R, Aripiprazole Study Group. Aripiprazole for treatment-resistant schizophrenia: results of a multicenter, randomized, double-blind, comparison study versus perphenazine. *J Clin Psychiatry.* 2007; 68(2): 213–23.

46   Holt RI, Peveler RC. Antipsychotics and hyperprolactinaemia: mechanisms, consequences and management. *Clin Endocrinol (Oxf).* 2011; 74(2): 141–7.

47 Stroup TS, Gray N. Management of common adverse effects of antipsychotic medications. *World Psychiatry*. 2018; 17(3): 341–56.

48 Kane JM, Correll CU, Goff DC, Kirkpatrick B, Marder SR, Vester-Blokland E, et al. A multicenter, randomized, double-blind, placebo-controlled, 16-week study of adjunctive aripiprazole for schizophrenia or schizoaffective disorder inadequately treated with quetiapine or risperidone monotherapy. *J Clin Psychiatry*. 2009; 70 (10): 1348–57.

49 Costa AM, Lima MS, Mari JdJ. A systematic review on clinical management of antipsychotic-induced sexual dysfunction in schizophrenia. *Sao Paulo Med J*. 2006; 124(5): 291–7.

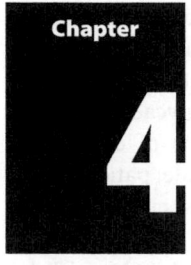

'Diabulimia', Diabetes and Eating Disorders

Anne M. Doherty, Aoife M. Egan and Seán F. Dinneen

Introduction

Eating disorders are common in diabetes and, where present, are associated with a much higher incidence of diabetic complications and a seven-fold increase in mortality (1). The comorbid presence of diabetes and an eating disorder can pose significant challenges to optimal management, and a multidisciplinary approach is key to reversing the poor outcomes associated with these conditions. The term 'diabulimia' is increasingly used by patient groups and in the general (and social) media. However, it is not a diagnostic term: there has been no professional agreement regarding what constitutes 'diabulimia' or what may constitute a minimum set of criteria for diagnosis.

Epidemiology and Risk

Anorexia nervosa has a prevalence of 0.3% in young women (peak age of onset 15–19 years) and it the deadliest of all mental disorders, with a crude mortality rate of 5.1 deaths/1,000 person-years (2). Bulimia nervosa has a prevalence of 1.0% in women and 0.1% in men, with an older age of onset than that of anorexia nervosa, and it has a crude mortality rate of 1.9 deaths/1,000 person-years (2). Binge-eating disorder has a prevalence of 1.9% in women and 0.3% in men and is associated with obesity (for further discussion of the relationship between obesity and mental health difficulties, see Chapter 10).

In addition, there are atypical presentations of eating disorder, variously typified as eating disorder not otherwise specified (EDNOS) and other specified feeding or eating disorder (OSFED). These are more common than the other eating disorders, with an estimated lifetime prevalence of 4.8% (3). These are often consider to be subclinical eating disorders, although in the presence of a comorbidity such as diabetes they may have quite serious consequences.

Patients who have a diagnosis of an eating disorder comorbid with diabetes are recognised as a highly complex patient group with high levels of excess morbidity and mortality compared with patients who have only one of these diagnoses, each of which in itself confers increased rates of morbidity and mortality (1). Eating disorders are up to four times more common in women than in men (4, 5). Eating disorders and subthreshold eating disorders are significantly more prevalent in female patients with type 1 diabetes compared to their peers without diabetes (3, 6–8). In particular, the practice of restricting insulin in order to achieve weight loss has been found to be a common behaviour among women with diabetes. In a study that examined the behaviours of 341 women with type 1 diabetes, Polonsky et al. found that 31% reported that they had a history of omitting insulin (9). Furthermore, the participating women also reported a greater incidence of disordered eating and fears of weight gain as a result of improved glycaemic control (9).

Patients with diabetes and an eating disorder have higher rates of hospital admission and unscheduled care (10). Good glycaemic control is difficult for patients with diabetes and disturbed eating behaviours to achieve in comparison to patients with normal eating patterns, and this results in a more negative prognosis overall (6). Poor glycaemic control has been associated with early onset of the microvascular complications of diabetes in women with type 1 diabetes (11). Goebel-Fabbri et al.'s study of female patients with diabetes found that at the 11-year follow-up insulin omission was associated with an increased mortality risk (12). Similarly, Nielsen et al.'s 10-year follow-up study found that the standardised mortality rate for people with type 1 diabetes was 2.5%, but it was 6.5% for people with anorexia nervosa and 34.8% in those with both conditions (1).

Diagnosing an Eating Disorder

Anorexia Nervosa

The diagnostic criteria for anorexia nervosa have been established in the two main diagnostic schedules: the *Diagnostic and Statistical Manual of Mental Disorders*, 5th edition (DSM-5) of American Psychiatric Association (APA) and the Tenth Revision of the International Classification of Disease and Related Health Problems (ICD-10) of the World Health Organization (WHO) (13, 14). There is agreement on the basic criteria: low body weight <17.5 kg/m^2, fear of fatness and body image disturbance. There are two recognised subtypes: restrictive and purging subtypes. The restrictive subtype is characterised in the main by an extreme restriction of dietary intake with the intention of maintaining a low body weight. The purging subtype includes symptoms and behaviours such as self-induced vomiting and the use of laxatives and diuretics. In type 1 diabetes, 'purging' may also occur by insulin omission with resultant glycosuria, calorie loss and an increased risk of ketoacidosis. The diagnostic criteria in ICD-10 and DSM-5 are compared in Table 4.1 (13, 14).

Bulimia Nervosa

In bulimia nervosa, like anorexia nervosa, there is a fear of weight gain. However, periods of starvation and restriction are counterbalanced by episodes of binge-eating. These binges are characteristically followed by periods of intense guilt about the binge and attempts to negate the weight gain by purging. Like in the purging subtype of anorexia nervosa, these attempts include self-induced vomiting and the use of laxatives and diuretics. Patients with bulimia nervosa often first present with the sequelae of purging, namely electrolyte disturbance.

Binge-Eating Disorder

Binge-eating disorder has the primary symptom of binge-eating of bulimia nervosa with few compensatory behaviours and is associated with obesity.

Other Eating Disorders

The atypical presentations of eating disorders, variously typified as EDNOS and OSFED, have some of the symptoms of the other eating disorders without meeting full diagnostic criteria (see Table 4.1).

Table 4.1 Diagnostic criteria for eating disorders.

	DSM-5	ICD-10
Anorexia nervosa	• Persistent restriction of energy intake leading to significantly low body weight • Either an intense fear of gaining weight or of becoming fat or persistent behaviour that interferes with weight gain • Disturbance of body image	• Body mass index <17.5 kg/m^2 • Dietary restriction and other weight loss efforts • Body image distortion • Amenorrhoea in women; loss of sexual interest and potency in men
Bulimia nervosa	• Recurrent episodes of binge-eating • Compensatory behaviours including vomiting, purging, starvation and misuse of medications • Binge-eating and compensatory behaviours occur (on average) once weekly for 3 months • Self-evaluation based on shape/size	• Episodes of overeating • Efforts to counteract overeating by vomiting, purging, starvation and misuse of medications • Morbid dread of fatness
Binge-eating disorder	• Recurrent episodes of binge-eating • Episodes characterised by distress regarding binge-eating • Binge-eating occurs on average once weekly for 3 months • Not associated with compensatory behaviours	Not included in ICD-10
Other	OSFED: Symptoms cause significant distress or impairment, but do not meet full criteria of conditions above Avoidant/restrictive food intake disorder (ARFID): Restricted intake limited to a narrow repertoire of foods, with avoidance based on appearance, texture, smell or other features	EDNOS: Some symptoms of the conditions but not to diagnostic threshold

Purging by Insulin Omission and Glycosuria

The practice of restricting insulin in order to achieve weight loss has been found to be a common behaviour among women with type 1 diabetes (10). This is functionally a form of purging, and it may be perceived by the person doing it as a simple method of achieving weight loss that does not require any specific acts (e.g. vomiting or taking medications), and one that results in poorer glycaemic control. It is thus a very passive and attractive form of purging in which there is no immediate reminder of the act and no immediate unpleasant physical sensation as there is in vomiting.

Patients who are trying to regulate weight with insulin omission will have suboptimal glycaemic control, reflected in high levels of HbA1c, and they may present with recurrent diabetic ketoacidosis (DKA). With a high index of suspicion for disordered eating, assessment of the patient with recurrent DKA should always include a discussion about weight and insulin omission and a referral onwards to liaison psychiatry, eating disorder psychiatry or the local community mental health team as appropriate.

Diagnostic Challenges

National Institute for Health and Care Excellence (NICE) guidelines state that patients with diabetes should be routinely screened for eating disorder, especially when there is poor adherence to treatment (15). However, this is difficult to implement in practice due to the difficulties in detection and the awareness of clinicians regarding local treatment options. It is also unethical to screen patients for a condition for which there is no available treatment or that existing services do not have the capacity to provide. Where there are eating disorder services available it should be possible for an individual with diabetes and a formal diagnosis of anorexia nervosa to access treatment. There may be difficulties, however, when the symptoms are atypical at the 'milder' end of bulimia nervosa or in the EDNOS category, where specialist eating disorder services may not be able to provide a service, especially if a screening programme results in a high volume of referrals.

In addition, patients known to have a diagnosis of eating disorder will frequently present with difficulties related to their diabetes, and it is important that eating disorder clinicians are comfortable with the management of these problems with the support of the diabetes team.

Management 1: General Principles in the Management of Eating Disorders

The three main areas of treatment of eating disorders are nutritional therapy and refeeding, psychological therapies and pharmacological treatments. The majority of eating disorder care is delivered in the community by specialist eating disorder services (or by general adult psychiatry teams where eating disorder services are not available). Treatment is tailored to the patients' needs and, depending on the severity of symptoms, stage of treatment and patient preference, they may be delivered in inpatient units, day hospital settings or outpatient clinics.

The mainstay of treatment is psychological therapy, with a strong evidence base for cognitive behavioural therapy (especially for bulimia nervosa) and family therapy (especially for anorexia nervosa and in younger patients). In the more severe stages of illness, it may be very difficult for patients to properly engage with psychological therapy: at these times, the focus is on supporting the optimisation of nutritional status.

Pharmacological treatments should not be used as the primary treatment of eating disorders, but rather as adjunctive treatments in bulimia nervosa or binge-eating disorder or to treat conditions comorbid with anorexia nervosa (15, 16).

Management 2: Severely Medically Unwell Patients with an Eating Disorder

People with anorexia nervosa have a high mortality rate and may present to hospital critically ill requiring medical admission. Despite being gravely ill, they may seem 'deceptively well' to those unfamiliar with the condition (17, 18). The reason for hospitalisation may take a number of forms, including electrolyte derangements, electrocardiogram changes or perhaps a very low body mass index (BMI) requiring urgent refeeding

Table 4.2 Modified MARSIPAN table.

System	Test/investigation	Moderate risk	High risk
Nutritional	Body mass index Rate of weight loss Glucose	<15 kg/m^2 >0.5 kg/week Concern if abnormal	<13 kg/m^2 or 70% of median for age if <18 years >1 kg/week for >2 weeks <3 mmol/L
Cardiovascular	BP Postural drop Pulse rate Oedema Peripheral cyanosis	$<90/60$ mmHg >10 mmHg <50 bpm Ankle or sacral oedema	$<80/50$ mmHg >15 mmHg <40 bpm Bilateral pitting oedema
Musculoskeletal	Stand up–squat test (lying on floor, sits up without using hands or sitting on chair, stands without using hands)	Grade 2 (able to rise with noticeable difficulty)	Grades 0–1 (unable to rise or able only to rise with the use of hands)
Temperature		$<35°C$	$<34.5°C$
Haematological	White cell count Neutrophils Haemoglobin Platelets	Concern if abnormal	$<2.0 \times 10^9$/L $<1.0 \times 10^9$/L <9.0 g/dL $<110 \times 10^9$/L
Biochemical	Potassium Sodium Phosphate	Concern if abnormal	<3 mmol/L <130 mmol/L <0.5 mmol/L
ECG	Pulse rate Corrected QT interval (QTc) Arrhythmias	<50 bpm	<40 bpm >450 ms Any arrhythmia

BP: blood pressure; ECG: electrocardiogram.

under supervision (to avoid the development of a refeeding syndrome), and refeeding may be oral feeding or nasogastric feeding. The Management of Really Sick Patients with Anorexia Nervosa (MARSIPAN) guidelines developed by a number of British Medical Royal Colleges are freely downloadable and are useful in managing these critical situations and allowing patients to be treated promptly and appropriately. They offer quite a prescriptive plan for the management of patients with a BMI of <15 kg/m^2. Many hospitals or trusts will have a local variant of the guidelines (outlined in Table 4.2) and in general either a consultant gastroenterologist or endocrinologist will lead on the care, in partnership with either a consultant psychiatrist specialist in eating disorders or a consultant in liaison psychiatry. Input from dietetics and mental health nursing is also required. The MARSIPAN guidelines explain the importance of constant supervision to minimise any behaviours that may threaten or undermine treatment gains and the importance of team communication. There is a similar document for the emergency medical treatment of children and adolescents with eating disorders: Junior MARSIPAN

(19). Other jurisdictions have similar documents to guide the management of patients requiring inpatient medical treatment (20, 21).

The MARSIPAN guidelines clarify the appropriateness of using mental health or capacity legislation where indicated and appropriate, bearing in mind the differing mental health legislation in different jurisdictions, even within the UK. MARSIPAN reiterates that a severe eating disorder is a life-threatening mental disorder for which treatment is, in the immediate term, feeding under careful supervision. Patients may require transfer to a psychiatric ward (preferably a specialist eating disorder unit) as soon as they can be safely discharged from a medical ward due to the importance of accessing medical and nursing expertise in the management of symptomatic behaviours and having access to the collective expertise of the multidisciplinary eating disorder team. Less critical medical issues such as derangements of thyroid or liver function may be followed up by the medical team when the patient is in a psychiatric/eating disorder unit or as an outpatient.

Management 3: Comorbid Diabetes and Eating Disorder

There may be challenges in adequately coordinating the care of this complex patient group on a case-by-case basis. These challenges (e.g. limited access to relevant clinical data) are currently overcome by the goodwill of individual clinicians. A preferred solution would be for the health system to facilitate a more integrated approach to care between the community, hospital and the multiple sub-specialities involved. Differing degrees of severity of illness will require different treatments and different settings, as outlined in Table 4.3.

A focus group examining the experiences of patients who have diabetes and eating disorders reported that multidisciplinary teamwork is very important in their recovery and that there is a need for patient involvement in the planning of care (22). Some have reported that perceived rigid or critical attitudes from professionals may even trigger a relapse of illness, indicating that further training in this complex area is required for the professionals involved.

In developing the NICE guidelines on eating disorders, particular consideration was given to whether patients with eating disorders required modified treatment where comorbid diabetes was present, considering the resource implications of integrated care. The conclusion reached was that while the limited evidence showed some support for modified treatment, the evidence was not adequate to support specific guidelines for diabetes and eating disorder (15). The Joint British Diabetes Societies (JBDS) and Royal College of Psychiatrists (RCPsych) guidelines recommend that the successful management of disordered eating in diabetes should include a number of key components, as outlined in the following subsections (23).

Monitoring

It is important to ensure routine monitoring for disordered eating among patients with diabetes, in particular to assess for insulin omission. This needs to be supported by staff who are comfortable asking about these topics (in a similar way to staff asking sensitively about pregnancy). In many cases, the clinician best situated to have these conversations may be the diabetes specialist nurse who has a long-term relationship with the patient, rather than a doctor in secondary care who may only meet the person once and may not have the same opportunities to develop a relationship of trust. There is evidence that secrecy around insulin omission may be important as a driver of a personal sense of 'empowerment', and

Table 4.3 Key components of the general management of eating disorders (EDs).

Setting[a]	Treatments	Key clinical staff
Medical inpatient	Stabilisation Refeeding MARSIPAN guideline-based care	Physician (often gastroenterologist, endocrinologist) Psychiatrist (liaison psychiatrist or eating disorder psychiatrist) Dietician Nursing staff
Inpatient eating disorder unit	Psychological therapies – CBT for EDs – Family therapy Nutritional therapy – Dietetics – Meal support Pharmacotherapy where indicated Physical heath monitoring	ED psychiatrist Psychology Specialist ED nursing ED dietician
Day hospital	Psychological therapies – CBT for EDs – Family therapy Nutritional therapy ● Dietetics ● Meal support Pharmacotherapy where indicated Physical heath monitoring	ED psychiatrist Psychology Specialist ED nursing ED dietician
Outpatient	Psychological therapies – CBT for EDs – Family therapy Nutritional therapy – Dietetics Pharmacotherapy where indicated Physical heath monitoring	ED psychiatrist Psychology ED dietician

[a] Settings are listed in order of level of severity, with those requiring medical inpatient treatment being the most severely ill and those in the outpatient setting being the least severely ill.
CBT: cognitive behavioural therapy.

where present, this may be an obstacle to the patient disclosing symptoms of eating disorder, highlighting the importance of having a trusting relationship with at least one member of the diabetes team (24). If screening for eating disorder does not occur, it is important to have a higher index of suspicion in patients with persistently elevated HbA1c, recurrent DKA and ketonuria. A simple dipstick test for ketosis may be a quick and easy way of identifying people who warrant further assessment.

Communication

Good communication between the professionals managing the eating disorder and those managing the diabetes is key in order to manage these risks and optimise prognosis. This may be via regular meetings or *ad hoc* communications. We need to ensure that we have an evidence-based pathway for the care of patients with this complex clinical picture. It is important that the relevant clinical information (both medical and psychiatric) is readily available to the clinicians involved in the care of individuals with these comorbidities in order to optimise their management (23).

Collaboration

Multidisciplinary management of patients with eating disorders and type 1 diabetes should include diabetes professionals attending multidisciplinary team meetings in eating disorder (or generic mental health) services (both inpatient and outpatient). Patients with type 1 diabetes and anorexia nervosa admitted to inpatient psychiatric units are at high risk of developing DKA, which is more common than refeeding syndrome. In addition to the theoretical risk of spontaneous hypoglycaemia and/or hypophosphataemia from the insulin stimulus, it may be difficult to achieve glycaemic control under optimal conditions (23).

Some authors have recommended 'permissive hyperglycaemia' in order to minimise these risks (25).

In view of the rarity of this occurrence and the psychiatric–medical complexity of these presentations, the JBDS and RCPsych guidelines recommend specialist diabetes input into the management of hyperglycaemia during refeeding in an eating disorder or general psychiatric facility (23).

Building Expertise: Staff Education and Training

This should begin with enhancing awareness of both eating disorders and disordered eating among diabetes clinicians and progress to developing confidence among members of the diabetes team in asking about insulin omission in a non-judgemental and sensitive manner. In addition, the identification and treatment of disordered eating will require clinicians to focus on behaviours such as insulin restriction and to explore with the patient their thoughts around weight and shape associated with insulin use. Finally, training in enhanced communication skills is needed to minimise the stigma that people with disordered eating perceive from clinicians and to avoid disengagement and drop out from clinical services (23).

Education of eating disorder services on the management of diabetes is likewise central to developing a collaborative approach to treatment. To date, there has been some work in enhanced diabetes education of eating disorders unit staff by the diabetes team and of the diabetes teams by specialists in eating disorders. This is usually informal and, where present, is often addressed on a case-by-case basis by joint working between the diabetes and eating disorders services, with some incidental cross-pollination of knowledge and skills. However, improved knowledge of both conditions and how they interact and improved skills in their optimal management are essential components of best practice.

In the absence of formal care pathways and with the segregation of clinical information, this can be a difficult and time-consuming task (23).

Screening and Centres of Excellence

Certain high-risk groups, such as transition services, may benefit from the use of routine screening, but only where there is a pathway for further management. The guidelines developed in the UK by the RCPsych and the JBDS recommend developing regional specialist centres of expertise in type 1 diabetes and eating disorders to build capacity, increase expertise, raise awareness, enable networking and produce consensus guidelines (23).

Care Pathways

There are no established pathways for the care of patients with diabetes and comorbid eating disorder. As a result, the management of such cases is *ad hoc*, unstandardised and variable. While bearing in mind the individual nature of the needs of these patients, it is important to ensure that the highest standards are met and that the organisations involved facilitate this process. This will frequently involve the close joint working of diabetes specialists with specialists in eating disorders and/or liaison psychiatry (23).

Additional Endocrine Manifestations: Bone and Reproductive Health

Reproductive and skeletal manifestations are commonly observed in those with eating disorders. These complications are mostly described in women with anorexia nervosa, but they can also occur in males and in those with bulimia nervosa (26). The low energy availability in women who restrict calories frequently results in hypothalamic amenorrhea and infertility (27). While recovery of reproductive function appears to be achievable when a 'critical body weight' is reached, there is no clear cut-off at which this occurs within an individual (28). Men may develop a similar endocrinopathy with low serum testosterone concentrations (29). This low oestrogen and testosterone secretion combined with decreased levels of nutritionally dependent hormones such as IGF-1 and leptin are important contributors to bone loss in anorexia nervosa (30). In this regard, measurement of bone mineral density using dual X-ray absorptiometry is important. A prospective cohort study of 130 women with anorexia nervosa identified osteopenia in 92% and osteoporosis in 38% (31). These abnormalities of bone density translate into a two- to three-fold increased fracture risk in both men and women, as demonstrated by a US-based longitudinal study (32).

Restoration of nutritional status is the cornerstone of therapy in affected patients. Particular emphasis should be placed on calcium and vitamin D supplementation to optimise bone health. Although weight-bearing exercise is generally considered beneficial to bone health, in the setting of an eating disorder this should be cautiously approached and highly individualised under expert supervision. Compulsive exercise is associated with eating disorders and while acutely ill excessive exercise may put patients at higher risk of hypogonadotropic hypogonadism, low bone mass and fracture. However, bone-loading activities have been shown to provoke bone accrual during recovery (33). Interestingly, high-dose oestrogen therapy (e.g. oral contraceptives) has not been shown to be effective for anorexia nervosa-associated bone loss (34). Some benefit is observed in adolescent girls treated with low-dose 'physiological' oestrogen replacement, and this approach is used in clinical practice (35). There are minimal data to support the use of therapies such as bisphosphonates or parathyroid hormone analogues; however, they may be useful in selected, more severe cases.

Conclusion

Eating disorders, while relatively rare, have the highest mortality rates of all mental disorders. When combined with diabetes, they have poor outcomes in terms of recurrent DKA, premature development of microvascular complications and mortality. It is important for endocrinologists to have a high index of suspicion for eating disorders in patients with diabetes (especially young women with type 1 diabetes). Psychiatrists need to consider and treat insulin omission as a form of purging in eating disorders. Overall, patients need joint management by psychiatrists and endocrinologists in close collaboration, with specialist input from dieticians, specialist nursing and specialist psychologists in order to optimise outcomes for people with these comorbidities.

References

1   Nielsen S, Emborg C, Mølbak AG. Mortality in concurrent type 1 diabetes and anorexia nervosa. *Diabetes Care*. 2002; 25: 309–12.

2   Arcelus J, Mitchell AJ, Wales J, Nielsen S. Mortality rates in patients 5 with anorexia nervosa and other eating disorders. A meta-analysis of 36 studies. *Arch Gen Psychiatry*. 2011: 68; 724–31.

3   Le Grange D, Lock J, Agras WS, Bryson SW, Jo B. A randomized clinical trial of family-based treatment and cognitive-behavioral therapy for adolescent bulimia nervosa. *J Am Acad Child Adolesc Psychiatry*. 2015; 54: 886–94.

4   Qian J, Hu Q, Wan Y, Li T, Wu M, Ren Z, et al. Prevalence of eating disorders in the general population: a systematic review. *Shanghai Arch Psychiatry*. 2013; 25: 212.

5   Hoek HW. Incidence, prevalence and mortality of anorexia nervosa and other eating disorders. *Curr Opin Psychiatry*. 2006; 19: 389–94.

6   Jones JM, Lawson ML, Daneman D, Olmsted MP, Rodin G. Eating disorders in adolescent females with and without type 1 diabetes: cross sectional study. *BMJ*. 2000; 320: 1563–6.

7   Ryan M, Gallanagh J, Livingstone MB, Gaillard C, Ritz P. The prevalence of abnormal eating behaviour in a representative sample of the French diabetic population. *Diabetes Metab*. 2008; 34: 581–6.

8   Olmsted MP, Colton PA, Daneman D, Rydall AC, Rodin GM. Prediction of the onset of disturbed eating behavior in adolescent girls with type 1 diabetes. *Diabetes Care*. 2008; 31: 1978–82.

9   Polonsky WH, Anderson BJ, Lohrer PA, Aponte JE, Jacobson AM, Cole CF. Insulin omission in women with IDDM. *Diabetes Care*. 1994; 17: 1178–85.

10 Goebel-Fabbri AE. Disturbed eating behaviors and eating disorders in type 1 diabetes: clinical significance and treatment recommendations. *Curr Diab Rep*. 2009; 9: 133–9.

11 Takii M, Uchigata Y, Tokunaga S, Amemiya N, Kinukawa N, Nozaki T, et al. The duration of severe insulin omission is the factor most closely associated with the microvascular complications of type 1 diabetic females with clinical eating disorders. *Int J Eat Disord*. 2008; 41: 259–64.

12 Goebel-Fabbri AE, Fikkan J, Franko DL, Pearson K, Anderson BJ, Weinger K. Insulin restriction and associated morbidity and mortality in women with type 1 diabetes. *Diabetes Care*. 2008; 31: 415–9.

13 APA. *The Diagnostic and Statistical Manual of Mental Disorders*

(5th ed. – DSM-5). American Psychiatric Publishing, 2013.

14 WHO. *The ICD-10 Classification of Mental and Behavioural Disorders: Clinical Descriptions and Diagnostic Guidelines.* World Health Organization, 1992.

15 NICE. Eating disorders: recognition and treatment, 2016. Available from: www.nice.org.uk/guidance/ng69

16 British Columbia Ministry for Health. Clinical Practice Guidelines for the BC Eating Disorders Continuum of Services, 2011. Available from: www.sisdca.it/public/pdf/BC-EATING-DISORDERS-CONTINUUM-OF-SERVICES-Clinical-Practice-Guidelines.pdf

17 Royal College of Psychiatrists, Royal College Physicians, Royal College of Pathologists. *MARSIPAN: Management of Really Sick Patients with Anorexia Nervosa* (2nd ed.) (College Report CR189). Royal College of Psychiatrists, 2014.

18 Jones WR, Morgan JF, Arcelus J. Managing physical risk in anorexia nervosa. *Adv Psychiatr Treat.* 2013; 19: 201–2.

19 Royal College of Psychiatrists, Royal College Physicians, Royal College of Pathologists. *Junior MARSIPAN: Management of Really Sick Patients under 18 with Anorexia Nervosa* (College Report CR168). Royal College of Psychiatrists, 2012.

20 Royal Australia and New Zealand College of Psychiatrists (RANZCP). Clinical Practice Guidelines for the Treatment of Eating Disorders (adult and child) (2014). Available from: www.ranzcp.org/files/resources/college_statements/clinician/cpg/eating-disorders-cpg.aspx

21 APA. Practice guideline for the treatment of patients with eating disorders, 2006. Available from: https://edsna.ca/wp-content/uploads/2017/07/apa_guideline_for_treatment_of_ed.pdf

22 Zaremba N, Watson A, Kan C, Broadley M, Partridge H, Figuereido C, et al. Multidisciplinary healthcare teams' challenges and strategies in supporting people with type 1 diabetes to recover from disordered eating. *Diabet Med.* 2020; 37: 1992–2000.

23 JBDS, RCPsych. The management if diabetes in adults and children with psychiatric disorders in inpatient settings, 2017. Available from: www.diabetes.org.uk/resources-s3/2017-10/Management%20of%20diabetes%20in%20adults%20and%20children%20with%20psychiatric%20disorders%20in%20inpatient%20settings-August-2017.pdf

24 Staite E, Zaremba N, Macdonald P, Allan J, Treasure J, Ismail K, Stadler M. 'Diabulima' through the lens of social media: a qualitative review and analysis of online blogs by people with type 1 diabetes mellitus and eating disorders. *Diabet Med.* 2018; 35: 1329–36.

25 Brown C, Mehler PS. Anorexia nervosa complicated by diabetes mellitus: the case for permissive hyperglycemia. *Int J Eat Disord.* 2014; 47: 671–4.

26 Kendall KA, Bulik CM, Joyce PR, McIntosh VV, Carter FA. Menstrual cycle irregularity in bulimia nervosa. Associated factors and changes with treatment. *J Psychosom Res.* 2000; 49: 409.

27 Schorr M, Miller KK. The endocrine manifestations of anorexia nervosa: mechanisms and management. *Nat Rev Endocrinol.* 2017; 13: 174–86.

28 Boyar RM, Katz J, Finkelstein JW, Kapen S, Weiner H, Weitzman ED, Hellman L. Anorexianervosa. Immaturity of the 2 hour luteinizing hormone secretory pattern. *N Engl J Med.*1974; 24: 861–5.

29 Skolnick A. Schulman RC, Galindo RJ, Mechanick JI. The endocrinopathies of male anorexia nervosa: case series. *AACE Clin Case Rep.* 2016; 2: e351–7.

30 Lawson EA,Klibanski A. Endocrine abnormalities in anorexia nervosa. *Nat Clin Pract Endocrinol Metab.* 2008; 4:407–14.

31 Grinspoon S,Thomas E,Pitts S,Gross E, Mickley D,Miller K,et al. Prevalence and predictive factors for regional osteopenia in women withanorexia nervosa. *Ann Intern Med.* 2000; 133: 790–4.

32 Lucas AR, Melton LJ 3rd,Crowson CS, O'Fallon WM. Long-term fracture risk among women withanorexia nervosa: a

population-based cohort study. *Mayo Clin Proc.*1999; 74: 972–7.

33   Waugh EJ,Woodside DB,Beaton DE,Coté P,Hawker GA. Effects of exercise on bone mass in young women with anorexia nervosa. *Med Sci Sports Exerc.*2011; 43: 755–63.

34   Golden NH, Lanzkowsky L, Schebendach J, Palestro CJ, Jacobson MS, Shenker IR. The

effect of estrogen–progestin treatment on bone mineral density in anorexia nervosa. *J Pediatr Adolesc Gynecol.* 2002; 15: 135.

35   Misra M, Katzman D, Miller KK, Mendes N, Snelgrove D, Russell M, et al. Physiologic estrogen replacement increases bone density in adolescent girls with anorexia nervosa. *J Bone Miner Res.* 2011; 26: 2430.

Disorders of the Hypothalamic–Pituitary–Adrenal Axis
Cushing's Syndrome and Beyond

Aoife M. Egan and Anne M. Doherty

Introduction

Stress occurs when our physiological and/or psychological homeostasis is threatened, or perceived to be so, by internal or external adverse forces (1). The primary endocrine effectors of the stress response are located in the paraventricular nucleus of the hypothalamus, the anterior lobe of the pituitary gland and the adrenal gland. These structures are referred to as the hypothalamic–pituitary–adrenal axis (HPA) (2). In the setting of stress, corticotrophin-releasing hormone (CRH) induces the release of adrenocorticotropic hormone (ACTH), which stimulates the synthesis and secretion of glucocorticoids from the adrenal gland (Figure 5.1). Glucocorticoids exert a wide range of effects and can influence cardiovascular function, immunity and inflammation, metabolism, reproduction and fluid volume (3). An important target organ is the brain, where glucocorticoids can affect neuronal differentiation and excitability, behavioural reactivity, mood and cognition (2, 4). This regulatory system works in conjunction with the sympatho-adrenal medullary (SAM) system, which releases catecholamines including noradrenaline and adrenaline. These systems are crucial to dealing with both physiological and psychological stress and restoring our steady state (5). Inappropriate regulation of the stress response has been linked to a wide array of pathologies, including hypertension, diabetes, osteoporosis and psychological disorders. In this chapter, we will focus on disorders of the HPA axis and their effects on mental health. This will include discussions on conditions associated with steroid excess and insufficiency. We will also describe the role of the HPA axis in primary mental health disorders.

Endogenous Cushing's Syndrome

Cushing's syndrome is a potentially lethal disorder characterised by excessive production of cortisol. The excess cortisol may be caused by either excess ACTH secretion (from a pituitary or other ectopic tumour) or independent adrenal overproduction of cortisol (6). The term 'Cushing's disease' is reserved for when the underlying cause is a pituitary tumour secreting excess ACTH. Manifestations of Cushing's syndrome can range from subclinical, cyclical and mild to rapid-onset presentations (7). The clinical features are very variable (Table 5.1) and many overlap with other conditions. However, once the condition is suspected clinically, biochemical testing should be performed. These tests are complex and must be individualised for each patient. They typically involve timed measurement of urine, serum or salivary cortisol at baseline or after administration of dexamethasone (6). When the HPA axis is functioning normally, any supraphysiological dose of dexamethasone will suppress pituitary ACTH secretion, and this will result in suppression of cortisol production from the adrenal glands. In Cushing's syndrome, the excess cortisol production

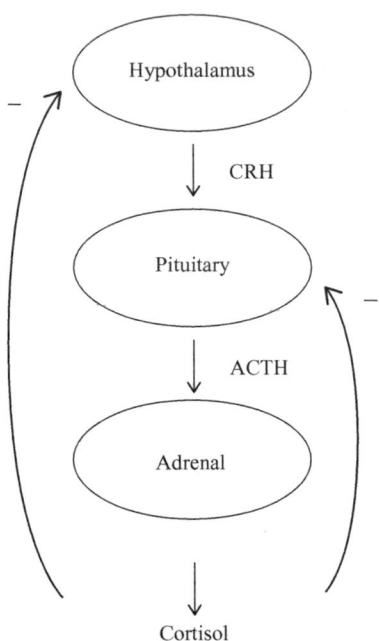

Figure 5.1 Hypothalamic–pituitary–adrenal (HPA) axis. ACTH: adrenocorticotropic hormone; CRH: corticotrophin-releasing hormone.

is typically not responsive to dexamethasone, hence the principle behind dexamethasone suppression testing. Once a diagnosis is established and the precise cause identified, surgical resection of the abnormal tissue is ideal. If this is not possible, medical therapy, radiation or bilateral adrenalectomy can be considered.

The first prospective study evaluating neuropsychiatric symptoms in active Cushing's syndrome included 35 patients (8). The authors reported a consistent constellation of psychiatric disturbances, including depressed mood (77%), irritability (86%), generalised anxiety (66%), increased crying (63%) and suicidal thoughts (17%). Social withdrawal (46%) was associated with shame about physical appearance and feelings of decreased focus. Some of these symptoms may be secondary to disturbed sleep, which was reported by a majority of patients, with 69% waking at least once during the night and 57% waking earlier than desired in the morning. In a separate study, researchers examined polysomnography profiles of patients with Cushing's syndrome, patients with major depressive disorder and healthy controls. Compared to healthy controls, the other groups demonstrated poorer sleep continuity, shortened rapid eye movement latency and increased first rapid eye movement period density (9). Cognitive symptoms associated with Cushing's syndrome include impaired memory (83%) and impaired concentration (66%) (10). Given the prevalence of neuropsychiatric symptoms, it is not surprising that a significant number of people with Cushing's syndrome meet criteria for a major depressive disorder. In 1985, Haskett obtained longitudinal psychiatric histories from 30 people with confirmed Cushing's syndrome due to tumours of the adrenal cortex and pituitary. Overall, 83% met diagnostic criteria for an episode of affective disorder during the course of their endocrine disturbance and 66% met criteria for endogenous depression (11). Depression during the active phase of Cushing's syndrome has been associated with older age, female sex, higher pretreatment

Table 5.1 Clinical features of Cushing's syndrome.

Weight gain
Central obesity
Supraclavicular/dorsocervical fat pads

Facial plethora
Facial rounding

Easy bruising
Acne
Hirsutism
Violaceous striae

Proximal muscle weakness
Osteopenia or osteoporosis

Hypertension
Glucose intolerance or diabetes mellitus
Dyslipidaemia
Decreased libido
Menstrual irregularity

Recurrent infections
Impaired wound healing

Headaches
Cataracts

Broad range of neuropsychiatric symptoms

urinary cortisol levels and past adverse life events (12). In patients with Cushing's disease specifically, major depression is associated with surgical failure, in addition to clinical features such as disease severity and lack of neuroradiological or surgical evidence of an adenoma (13).

As patients may not spontaneously mention neuropsychiatric symptoms, it is important to specifically enquire into this. Features such as irritability and adrenergic stimulation (e.g. shaking and increased sweating) may be more prominent in Cushing's syndrome compared to a primary major depressive disorder (14). It would also appear that pharmacotherapy such as tricyclic antidepressants or selective serotonin reuptake inhibitors have limited effectiveness, and the most effective approach is treatment of the hypercortisolism.

Patients in Remission from Cushing's Syndrome

Using the Symptom Checklist-90 questionnaire, Dorn et al. evaluated 33 patients with confirmed Cushing's syndrome. Before treatment, 66.7% of the patients had significant psychopathology – 51.5% with atypical depressive disorder and/or major affective disorder in 12%. The overall psychopathology decreased to 53.6% at 3 months, 36.0% at 6 months and 21.1% at 12 months following correction of the hypercortisolaemia and parallel recovery of the HPA axis (15). Sonino et al. noted that approximately 70% of patients with Cushing's syndrome recovered from depression following endocrine cure with no differences between patients with pituitary-dependent or pituitary-independent disease (16). However, among the remaining 30%, some patients reported no improvement in depression following cure of their Cushing's syndrome. Finally, Starkman et al. reported that 72% of patients with depressed mood experienced improvement after endocrine cure, 80% reported increased concentration and 70% reported an improvement of memory issues (8). The magnitude of decrease in urinary free cortisol correlates to improvement in depressed mood (17). Furthermore, as seen in those with a primary depressive disorder, features such as irritability and sleep disturbance may recover quickly with cortisol lowering; however, depressed mood may take longer to improve (14). It should be noted that although significant improvements in neuropsychiatric symptoms can be expected following treatment, patients with Cushing's syndrome frequently have persistent adverse effects. The experience of a cohort of patients who underwent definitive treatment for Cushing's disease within a 15-year period exemplifies this. Compared to those with other types of pituitary tumour, participants with Cushing's disease had significantly impaired psychological well-being and psychosocial functioning as measured by multiple psychological rating scales (18). Limited brain imaging studies correlate with clinical findings and reveal that in patients with active Cushing's disease, hippocampal volume is negatively correlated with plasma cortisol (19). Following treatment for the underlying endocrine disorder, there was a significant increase in hippocampal volume (20). However, re-imaging of patients with Cushing's syndrome several years after treatment reveals that measures of brain volume, although improved, remained different from those of control subjects (21). Valassi et al. attempted to identify associations between biochemical parameters and affective alterations after long-term Cushing's syndrome remission. They reported that delay to diagnosis was associated with depressive symptoms, and low serum concentrations of brain-derived neurotrophic factor (BDNF) were associated with more anxiety, depression and stress. BDNF is involved in HPA regulation and is highly expressed in areas of the brain controlling mood and stress (22). A number of patients will develop hypopituitarism following treatment for Cushing's disease. This is associated with a higher prevalence of psychiatric disturbance, including major depression and dysthymia, than what could be attributed solely to the presence of a chronic disorder (23). Patients with treated Cushing's disease therefore require long-term follow-up with appropriate referral for psychiatric and psychological assistance as required. In this setting, antidepressants may play a role in long-term therapy (14).

Exogenous Glucocorticoids

In 1950, Drs Edward C. Kendall and Philip S. Hench (Mayo Clinic, USA) and Dr Tadeus Reichstein (Basel University, Switzerland) were awarded the Nobel Prize in Physiology or Medicine (24). Their work resulted in the isolation of cortisone (which they termed Compound E) and its use in the treatment of rheumatoid arthritis. Today, glucocorticoids are in widespread clinical use due to their potent anti-inflammatory and immune-modulating effects. A population-based study using data from the French reimbursement healthcare system found that the prevalence of oral glucocorticoid use ranged from 14.7% to 17.1% in the years 2007–2014 (25). However, despite their important benefits, glucocorticoids are associated with multiple adverse effects, both physical and psychiatric (26).

The earliest case reports noted positive affective symptoms such as mood elevation, euphoria and a feeling of well-being. However, more concerning symptoms soon became evident (27). To date, there is substantial variability in the reported incidence of glucocorticoid-associated adverse psychiatric reactions (1.8–57.0%) in exposed patients. This is understandable given the wide range of doses, varying durations of therapy and differing patient populations (26). In addition, effects can range from mild cognitive changes to more extreme presentations with delirium, dementia or even steroid-induced psychoses with associated hallucinations, delusions and thought impairment.

Naber et al. evaluated 50 ophthalmological patients previously free of psychiatric symptoms and reported that 26% developed mania and 10% developed depression within three days of initiating therapy with high-dose methylprednisolone or fluocortolone (28). Brown et al. examined 32 patients with asthma receiving bursts of prednisone (>40 mg/ day) and found that there were significant increases from baseline on a mania scale with no increase in depression measures during the first three to seven days of prednisone therapy. Interestingly, those with past or current symptoms of depression had a significant decrease in depressive symptoms during prednisone therapy. When patients were reassessed after therapy discontinued (within two weeks or less), the measures had returned to baseline (29). Longer-term steroid use appears to be associated with more depressive than manic symptoms. For example, a study following 20 patients receiving prednisone therapy (7.5 mg/day) for six months found that depressive symptom severity was greater in the patients receiving prednisone compared to a group of 14 controls. In total, 60% of the steroid-treated patients met diagnostic criteria for a lifetime prednisone-induced mood disorder (30). Cognitive disturbances including difficulties of concentration and in retaining information are frequently reported in patients using long-term glucocorticoids, and although they are generally reversible, they may persist for years after steroid exposure (14, 31).

The dose of glucocorticoid appears to be the most important risk factor for the development of psychiatric symptoms (26). This is exemplified by data from the Boston Collaborative Drug Surveillance Program that show that 1.3% of those receiving 40 mg/day or less of prednisone had psychiatric disturbance compared to 4.6% of those receiving 41–80 mg/day. Among those receiving more than 80 mg/day, 18.4% had severe psychiatric presentations, including psychosis (32). Women seem to be at a higher risk than men for developing psychiatric symptoms, but age, prior exposure experiences or history of psychiatric illness do not appear to play a role (26, 33, 34).

As individual responses can be variable, providing patient education on the most commonly encountered potential adverse effects is important at the time of glucocorticoid initiation. Small case series do report successful use of a wide variety of prophylactic regimens, including lithium carbonate, chlorpromazine, valproic acid, gabapentin and lamotrigine (26). However, such prophylactic regimens are not typically used in clinical practice. Providers should therefore enquire about new psychiatric symptoms at each clinical review and encourage early intervention for any reactions (26). The most effective treatment is discontinuation of glucocorticoid therapy or tapering if this is not possible. The exact approach will depend on the severity of the symptoms and the underlying medical disorder. If the presentation is severe (such as the situation of steroid-induced psychosis) and additional pharmacological therapy is required, atypical antipsychotics such as olanzapine appear to be rapidly effective at doses from 2.5 to 20 mg/day (35). Antidepressants may be helpful in depressed patients who require long-term steroids, but they have the potential to exacerbate agitation and psychosis (26). Although corticosteroid dose reduction or withdrawal forms the cornerstone of therapy for associated psychiatric reactions, rapid dose reductions in patients receiving long-term or high-dose steroids can also trigger new psychiatric symptoms, and so tapering rather than abrupt withdrawal is advised if possible. Following on from this point, it is worth emphasising that administration of exogenous glucocorticoids can suppress the endogenous HPA axis, and when these steroids are discontinued, tertiary adrenal insufficiency can ensue. Tapering regimens are designed to avoid this and facilitate gradual recovery of the adrenal axis. There is little evidence to support any specific tapering regimen. However, while short-term glucocorticoid therapy (up to three weeks) can generally be stopped without a taper (or using a quick taper), a very gradual dose reduction (5–10% every one to four weeks) should be used in those receiving long-term glucocorticoids, with a goal of avoiding the symptoms and signs of cortisol deficiency due to HPA suppression. Testing for HPA axis function can occur when the patient is using 5 mg/day or less of prednisolone, prednisone or equivalent glucocorticoid (36). This typically warrants endocrinology specialist input and involves assessment of the early morning serum cortisol and/or 1 mg ACTH stimulation test. Of course, in any particular individual, the ability to taper glucocorticoids will also be dictated by the underlying disease and the need to avoid recurrent activity while using the minimum glucocorticoid dose to avoid unwanted Cushingoid side effects.

Anabolic–Androgenic Steroid Misuse

Anabolic–androgenic steroids (AASs) refer to synthetic variants of the male sex hormone testosterone. Anabolic effects include increased protein synthesis, muscle growth and erythropoiesis and androgenic effects include an increase in male traits such as facial hair and a deeper voice (37). Although in many jurisdictions the possession or sale of anabolic steroids without a valid prescription is illegal, misuse of AASs is common, especially among professional and recreational athletes (38). A survey of 1.1 million Americans revealed that 0.5% of the adult population said that they had ever used anabolic steroids, and in the 18–34-year-old age group approximately 1% had ever used anabolic steroids (38). Common orally administered anabolic steroids include oxymetholone, oxandrolone, methandrostenolone and stanozolol. Injectable options include nandrolone, decanoate, nandrolone and phenpropionate (39). The primary motivating factors behind AAS use are to enhance performance and to improve physical appearance (40). This approach is distinctly different from the use of physiological doses of sex hormones in the setting of an endocrine deficiency. When used at supraphysiological doses, these substances are associated with a multitude of undesirable consequences, including cardiovascular effects such as hypertension and dyslipidaemia. One can typically observe suppression of the endogenous production of gonadotropins and testosterone, and this can persist for an extended period of time after withdrawal (37). Gynaecomastia may occur due to peripheral conversion of androgens to oestradiol and oestrone, and acne and male pattern baldness are also observed. In women, clitoral hypertrophy, menstrual abnormalities and additional masculinising effects are frequent (39).

Misuse of AASs may lead to changes in behaviour, including increased aggression, hostility and lack of impulse control. 'Roid rage' refers to the sudden aggressive AAS-induced response to minimal provocation (40, 41). A study by Choi and Pope investigated the association between AAS use and domestic violence and found that users reported significantly more verbal aggression and violence against their female partners when taking the drugs (42). The connection between mood disorders and AAS misuse is well described; however, studies report significant variation in the severity of symptoms. One study comparing 88 athletes who were using AAS with 68 non-users identified that 23% reported major mood syndromes including mania, hypomania or major depression in association with their use compared to 6% in non-users (41). Another study examining mood alterations in male weightlifters found that AAS users scored higher on depression and mania rating scales, but no subjects met diagnostic criteria for a mood disorder (43). There is also concern that mood disorders may persist after cessation of the AAS use. This was suggested by a study of Swedish male elite power sport athletes who were former AAS users but experienced ongoing high rates of depressive symptomatology (44). Any form of substance abuse is a risk factor for suicide, and AAS misuse is not an exception. A prospective study of 62 Finnish male elite weightlifters with suspected AAS use identified a 4.6-times higher mortality rate compared to a control sample from the general population (n = 1,094) (45). In the AAS group, mortality was predominantly due to suicide and myocardial infarction. Greater social physique anxiety is associated with more severe symptoms of both AAS dependence and depression (46). In fact, athletes are frequently affected by somatoform and eating disorders. There is a similarity in the psychological profiles of people with anorexia and bodybuilders, with both groups exhibiting unhealthy behaviours including food restriction and extreme exercise (40, 47). Interestingly, bodybuilders report a positive self-image, which differs from those with anorexia. Anxiety disorders also appear to be more common in AAS users compared to non-users (12.0% versus 2.6%), as reported by a study examining the characteristics of 67 male AAS users compared to 76 male non-users. In this study, subjects ≥40 years of age were recruited through fitness, weightlifting, bodybuilding and steroid websites (48). Finally, psychotic reactions to AASs are described in a study of 41 bodybuilders and footballers taking AAS drugs, reporting a 12% prevalence of psychotic symptoms (49).

Overall, it is clear that misuse of AASs can be detrimental to mental health. Providers should take care to caution users regarding potential side effects and encourage discontinuation of the AASs. Ongoing psychological support and a medically supervised detoxification may be useful depending on the clinical circumstances and extent of the substance misuse (40). Depending on local availability, affected individuals would likely benefit from ongoing engagement with a substance misuse service. Abrupt discontinuation has the potential to trigger severe psychological symptoms, similar to the scenario of exogenous glucocorticoid use (50).

Addison's Disease

Addison's disease or primary adrenal insufficiency results from insufficient or absent production of steroid hormones from the adrenal cortex. In the past, tuberculosis leading to adrenal destruction was the most common aetiology; however, autoimmune adrenalitis is now the most frequent cause. Other infectious diseases, metastatic disease, certain medications, adrenal haemorrhage or infarction may also result in this condition (51). The presenting signs and symptoms of primary adrenal insufficiency are variable and non-specific (Table 5.2) and the diagnosis can often be delayed. Although the recent literature gives little attention to the psychiatric features, when Thomas Addison first described the disease in 1855, he noted that patients could develop 'Attacks of giddiness', 'anxiety in the

Table 5.2 Clinical features of primary adrenal insufficiency.

Fatigue
Weight loss
Anorexia
Muscle weakness
Hyperpigmentation (particularly in skin creases, mucosal membranes)
Nausea, vomiting, diarrhoea
Salt craving
Orthostatic hypotension
Broad range of psychiatric symptoms

face' and 'delirium' (52, 53). Anglin and colleagues summarised 25 cases of Addison's disease where neuropsychiatric symptoms were reported. Within this selected group, there was a high prevalence of delusions (56%), hallucinations (40%), depression (44%), irritability/aggression (24%) and anxiety (24%). Less commonly reported were symptoms of disorientation, memory impairment, mania and, rarely, catatonia and self-injury (53). In the majority of cases (80%), symptoms resolved rapidly with cortisone treatment, but they occasionally persisted for months. Although not well described, it is likely that psychiatric symptoms may also occur in secondary (impaired/absent ACTH production from the pituitary) or tertiary (hypothalamic abnormalities impairing CRH secretion) adrenal insufficiency. Appropriate hormone replacement forms the mainstay of treatment, and the introduction of psychotropic medications should be considered on a case-by-case basis only.

The HPA Axis in Mental Health Disorders

Over the course of the twentieth century, the relationship between stress and psychiatric disorders has become better understood. In addition to the development of the science of the autonomic stress response, central to this understanding has been a large body of work in the area of the HPA axis, which has encompassed its role in providing biomarkers of the stress response and as a mediator of the secondary physiological changes. The HPA axis, along with the locus coeruleus–norepinephrine system and, by extension, the central nervous system, are central to the physiology of stress, and disruption of these pathways may be associated with pathological manifestations of stress, including mood disorders (54). In response to stress, the HPA axis is activated following adrenal epinephrine secretion in response to activation of the autonomic sympathetic axis.

There is evidence that there may be significant differences in the HPA axis responses to stress in different phenotypes of depression (e.g. in melancholic or endogenous depression compared with atypical depression). Both subtypes have quite different symptoms: atypical depression is characterised by a reversal of the biological symptoms of endogenous depression instead of the classical reduced appetite, weight and sleep of endogenous depression. These subtypes have differing responses to treatment. Studies have demonstrated HPA axis overactivity in the more endogenous depressive subtypes, and atypical depression is characterised instead by hypocortisolism and an exaggerated negative feedback (55). Bipolar affective disorder is similarly associated with dysregulation of the HPA axis, and there is evidence that this may be stimulated by environmental rather than genetic factors (56).

The elevated plasma cortisol concentrations associated with depression can overlap with the range seen in Cushing's syndrome (57). In fact, when dexamethasone is administered to evaluate the sensitivity of the hypothalamus to feedback signals for the shutdown of CRH release, the normal suppression response of cortisol is absent in approximately half of severely depressed patients (58). In clinical practice, this can cause false positives when using the dexamethasone suppression test to evaluate for Cushing's syndrome, resulting in a diagnosis of 'pseudo-Cushing's syndrome'. Interestingly, it appears that when antidepressants are used to induce clinical remission from the depression, a reversal of the HPA disturbance may occur (57, 58). However, while CRH receptor antagonists have shown antidepressant activity in animal studies (59), results in humans have been disappointing (58). Although people with pseudo-Cushing's syndrome do not tend to have the classic signs of hypercortisolism on clinical examination, it is unclear whether the hypercortisolaemia present in persons with depression contributes to the increase in cardiovascular disease observed in this population.

The comorbidity of depression and irritable bowel syndrome resulted in an increase in focus on the relationship between the brain and the gut, and this has led to a growing body of science of the relationship between gut microbiota and mood, implicating the HPA axis (60). The most recent evidence suggests that the gut may play an important role in the development of dysregulation of the HPA axis, and animal models suggest that there may be a number of mechanisms whereby gut microbiota influence the HPA axis (61, 62). Elevations in interferon-alpha and IL-6 cytokines inhibit the negative feedback regulation mechanisms of the HPA axis, resulting in chronic hypercortisolaemia in chronic stress, which will ultimately reduce the sensitivity of immune cells to feedback (63). Thus, dietary management of neuroinflammation may be a potential target for preventing and treating depression (64) .

Adrenal Function: Additional Issues to Consider

It is prudent to mention the term 'adrenal fatigue' as it has received significant attention from healthcare professionals, patients and the popular media in recent years. This is based on the theory that chronic exposure to stressful situations can lead to overuse and functional failure of the adrenal glands, with symptoms of adrenal insufficiency. Neurasthenia, a syndrome characterised by lassitude, fatigue, headache and irritability, is commonly reported in this setting. Although adrenal insufficiency is diagnosed using blood tests, there is no test to diagnose adrenal fatigue (65). It is clearly important that patients presenting with such symptoms are evaluated thoroughly, with testing for conditions such as adrenal insufficiency, obstructive sleep apnoea and depression as indicated. However, at the time of writing, there is no clear evidence that adrenal fatigue exists as an entity (66), and we do not recommend glucocorticoid therapy for this indication.

Conclusions

Endogenous and exogenous glucocorticoids exert a wide range of biological effects, and when normal physiology is disrupted, unwanted side effects are common. These include psychological symptoms, which may have an abrupt and extreme presentation. Those at risk should be identified and receive education to facilitate the early identification and management of such symptoms. Restoration of normal homeostasis forms the cornerstone of treatment, with the addition of psychotropic agents in individual cases. AAS misuse is relatively common and is associated with a range of unwanted side effects, from behaviour change to psychosis. Persons misusing AASs require education, support and possibly medical detoxification. Finally, an interesting body of evidence links the HPA axis and a variety of mental health disorders, and clinicians should enquire about a diagnosis of depression and depressive symptoms when evaluating for Cushing's syndrome.

References

1   Charmandari E, Tsigos C, Chrousos G. Endocrinology of the stress response. *Annu Rev Physiol.* 2005; 67: 259–84.

2   Smith SM, Vale WW. The role of the hypothalamic–pituitary–adrenal axis in neuroendocrine responses to stress. *Dialogues Clin Neurosci.* 2006; 8(4): 383–95.

3   Sapolsky RM, Romero LM, Munck AU. How do glucocorticoids influence stress responses? Integrating permissive, suppressive, stimulatory, and preparative actions. *Endocr Rev.* 2000; 21 (1): 55–89.

4   Koning A-SCAM, Buurstede JC, van Weert LTCM, Meijer OC. Glucocorticoid and mineralocorticoid receptors in the brain: a transcriptional perspective. *J Endocr Soc.* 2019; 3(10): 1917–30.

5   Turner AI, Smyth N, Hall SJ, Torres SJ, Hussein M, Jayasinghe SU, et al. Psychological stress reactivity and future health and disease outcomes: a systematic review of prospective evidence. *Psychoneuroendocrinology.* 2020; 114: 104599.

6   Nieman LK. Recent updates on the diagnosis and management of Cushing's syndrome. *Endocrinol Metab (Seoul).* 2018; 33(2): 139–46.

7   Lacroix A, Feelders RA, Stratakis CA, Nieman LK, et al. Cushing's syndrome. *Lancet.* 2015; 386(9996): 913–27.

8   Starkman MN, Schteingart DE, Schork MA. Depressed mood and other psychiatric manifestations of Cushing's syndrome: relationship to hormone levels. *Psychosom Med.* 1981; 43(1): 3–18.

9   Shipley JE, Schteingart DE, Tandon R, Pande AC, Grunhaus L, Haskett RF, Starkman MN. EEG sleep in Cushing's disease and Cushing's syndrome: comparison with patients with major depressive disorder. *Biol Psychiatry.* 1992; 32(2): 146–55.

10 Starkman MN, Schteingart DE, Schork MA. Correlation of bedside cognitive and neuropsychological tests in patients with Cushing's syndrome. *Psychosomatics.* 1986; 27(7): 508–11.

11 Haskett RF. Diagnostic categorization of psychiatric disturbance in Cushing's syndrome. *Am J Psychiatry.* 1985; 142(8): 911–6.

12 Santos A, Resmini E, Pascual JC, Crespo I, Webb SM. Psychiatric symptoms in patients with Cushing's syndrome: prevalence, diagnosis and management. *Drugs.* 2017; 77(8): 829–42.

13 Sonino N, Zielezny M, Fava GA, Fallo F, Boscaro M. Risk factors and long-term outcome in pituitary-dependent Cushing's disease. *J Clin Endocrinol Metab.* 1996; 81 (7): 2647–52.

14 Starkman MN. Neuropsychiatric findings in Cushing syndrome and exogenous glucocorticoid administration. *Endocrinol Metab Clin North Am.* 2013; 42 (3): 477–88.

15 Dorn LD, Burgess ES, Friedman TC, Dubbert B, Gold PW, Chrousos GP. The longitudinal course of psychopathology in Cushing's syndrome after correction of hypercortisolism. *J Clin Endocrinol Metab.* 1997; 82(3): 912–9.

16 Sonino N, Fava GA, Belluardo P, Girelli ME, Boscaro M. Course of depression in Cushing's syndrome: response to treatment and comparison with Graves' disease. *Horm Res.* 1993; 39(5–6): 202–6.

17 Starkman MN, Schteingart DE, Schork MA. Cushing's syndrome after treatment: changes in cortisol and ACTH levels, and amelioration of the depressive syndrome. *Psychiatry Res.* 1986; 19(3): 177–88.

18 Heald AH, Ghosh S, Bray S, Gibson C, Anderson SG, Buckler H, Fowler HL. Long-term negative impact on quality of life in patients with successfully treated Cushing's disease. *Clin Endocrinol (Oxf).* 2004; 61(4): 458–65.

19 Starkman MN, Gebarski SS, Berent S, Schteingart DE. Hippocampal formation volume, memory dysfunction, and cortisol levels in patients with Cushing's syndrome. *Biol Psychiatry.* 1992; 32(9): 756–65.

20 Starkman MN, Giordani B, Gebarski SS, Berent S, Schork MA, Schteingart DE. Decrease in cortisol reverses human hippocampal atrophy following treatment of Cushing's disease. *Biol Psychiatry.* 1999; 46(12): 1595–602.

21 Bourdeau I, Bard C, Forget H, Boulanger Y, Cohen H, Lacroix A. Cognitive function and cerebral assessment in patients who have Cushing's syndrome. *Endocrinol Metab Clin North Am.* 2005; 34(2): 357–69, ix.

22 Valassi E, Crespo I, Keevil BG, Aulinas A, Urgell E, Santos A, et al. Affective alterations in patients with Cushing's syndrome in remission are associated with decreased BDNF and cortisone levels. *Eur J Endocrinol.* 2017; 176(2): 221–31.

23 Lynch S, Merson S, Beshyah SA, Skinner E, Sharp P, Priest RG, Johnston DG. Psychiatric morbidity in adults with hypopituitarism. *J R Soc Med.* 1994; 87(8): 445–7.

24 The 1950 Nobel Prize in Physiology or Medicine. *Mayo Clin Proc.* 2000; 75(12): 1232.

25 Bénard-Laribière A, Pariente A, Pambrun E, Bégaud B, Fardet L, Noize P. Prevalence and prescription patterns of oral glucocorticoids in adults: a retrospective cross-sectional and cohort analysis in France. *BMJ Open.* 2017; 7(7): e015905.

26 Warrington TP, Bostwick JM. Psychiatric adverse effects of corticosteroids. *Mayo Clin Proc.* 2006; 81(10): 1361–7.

27 Sirois F. Steroid psychosis: a review. *Gen Hosp Psychiatry.* 2003; 25(1): 27–33.

28 Naber D, Sand P, Heigl B. Psychopathological and neuropsychological effects of 8-days' corticosteroid treatment. A prospective study. *Psychoneuroendocrinology.* 1996; 21 (1): 25–31.

29 Brown ES, Suppes T, Khan DA, Carmody 3rd TJ. Mood changes during prednisone bursts in outpatients with asthma. *J Clin Psychopharmacol.* 2002; 22(1): 55–61.

30 Bolanos SH, Khan DA, Hanczyc M, Bauer MS, Dhanani N, Brown ES. Assessment of mood states in patients receiving long-term corticosteroid therapy and in controls with patient-rated and clinician-rated scales. *Ann Allergy Asthma Immunol.* 2004; 92(5): 500–5.

31 Wolkowitz OM, Lupien SJ. Bigler ED. The 'steroid dementia syndrome': a possible model of human glucocorticoid neurotoxicity. *Neurocase.* 2007; 13(3): 189–200.

32 Acute adverse reactions to prednisone in relation to dosage. *Clin Pharmacol Ther.* 1972; 13(5): 694–8.

33 Stiefel FC, Breitbart WS, Holland JC. Corticosteroids in cancer: neuropsychiatric complications. *Cancer Invest.* 1989; 7(5): 479–91.

34 Ling MH, Perry PJ, Tsuang MT. Side effects of corticosteroid therapy. Psychiatric aspects. *Arch Gen Psychiatry.* 1981; 38(4): 471–7.

35 Brown ES, Varghese FP, McEwen BS. Association of depression with medical illness: does cortisol play a role? *Biol Psychiatry.* 2004; 55(1): 1–9.

36 Furst DE, Saag K. *Glucocorticoid withdrawal,* 2019. Available from: www .uptodate.com/contents/glucocorticoid-withdrawal

37 Hartgens F, Kuipers H. Effects of androgenic–anabolic steroids in athletes. *Sports Med.* 2004; 34(8): 513–54.

38 US Department of Justice Drug Enforcement Administration. A Guide for Understanding Steroids and Related Substances, 2004. Available from: www .deadiversion.usdoj.gov/pubs/brochures/ steroids/professionals

39 Maravelias C, Dona A, Stefanidou M, Spiliopoulou C. Adverse effects of anabolic steroids in athletes. A constant threat. *Toxicol Lett.* 2005; 158(3): 167–75.

40 Piacentino D, Kotzalidis GD, del Casale A, Aromatario MR, Pomara C, Girardi P, Sani G. Anabolic–androgenic steroid use and psychopathology in athletes. A systematic review. *Curr Neuropharmacol.* 2015; 13(1): 101–21.

41 Pope HG, Katz DL. Psychiatric and medical effects of anabolic–androgenic steroid use. A controlled study of 160 athletes. *Arch Gen Psychiatry.* 1994; 51(5): 375–82.

42 Choi PY, Pope HG. Violence toward women and illicit androgenic–anabolic steroid use. *Ann Clin Psychiatry.* 1994; 6(1): 21–5.

43 Perry PJ, Kutscher EC, Lund BC, Yates WR, Holman TL, Demers L. Measures of aggression and mood changes in male weightlifters with and without androgenic anabolic steroid use. *J Forensic Sci.* 2003; 48 (3): 646–51.

44 Lindqvist AS, Moberg T, Eriksson BO, Ehrnborg C, Rosén T, Fahlke C. A retrospective 30-year follow-up study of former Swedish-elite male athletes in power sports with a past anabolic androgenic steroids use: a focus on mental health. *Br J Sports Med.* 2013; 47(15): 965–9.

45 Pärssinen M, Kujala U, Vartiainen E, Sarna S, Seppälä T. Increased premature mortality of competitive powerlifters suspected to have used anabolic agents. *Int J Sports Med.* 2000; 21(3): 225–7.

46 Griffiths S, Jacka B, Degenhardt L, Murray SB, Larance B. Physical appearance concerns are uniquely associated with the severity of steroid dependence and depression in anabolic–androgenic steroid

users. *Drug Alcohol Rev.* 2018; 37(5): 664–70.

47 Davis C, Scott-Robertson L. A psychological comparison of females with anorexia nervosa and competitive male bodybuilders: body shape ideals in the extreme. *Eat Behav.* 2000; 1(1): 33–46.

48 Ip EJ, Trinh K, Tenerowicz MJ, Pal J, Lindfelt TA, Perry PJ. Characteristics and behaviors of older male anabolic steroid users. *J Pharm Pract.* 2015; 28(5): 450–6.

49 Pope HG, Katz DL. Affective and psychotic symptoms associated with anabolic steroid use. *Am J Psychiatry.* 1988; 145(4): 487–90.

50 Brower KJ, Blow FC, Beresford TP, Fuelling C. Anabolic–androgenic steroid dependence. *J Clin Psychiatry.* 1989; 50(1): 31–3.

51 Chabre O, Goichot B, Zenaty D, Bertherat J. Group 1. Epidemiology of primary and secondary adrenal insufficiency: prevalence and incidence, acute adrenal insufficiency, long-term morbidity and mortality. *Ann Endocrinol (Paris).* 2017; 78 (6): 490–4.

52 Addison T. *On the Constitutional and Local Effects of Disease of the Suprarenal Capsules.* Classics of Medicine Library, 1980.

53 Anglin RE, Rosebush PI, Mazurek MF. The neuropsychiatric profile of Addison's disease: revisiting a forgotten phenomenon. *J Neuropsychiatry Clin Neurosci.* 2006; 18 (4): 450–9.

54 Shelton RC. The molecular neurobiology of depression. *Psychiatr Clin North Am.* 2007; 30(1): 1–11.

55 Juruena MF, Bocharova M, Agustini B, Young AH. Atypical depression and non-atypical depression: Is HPA axis function a biomarker? A systematic review. *J Affect Disord.* 2018; 233: 45–67.

56 Belvederi Murri M, Prestia D, Mondelli V, Pariante C, Patti S, Olivieri B, et al. The HPA axis in bipolar disorder: systematic review and meta-analysis. *Psychoneuroendocrinology.* 2016; 63: 327–42.

57 Carroll BJ, Cassidy F, Naftolowitz D, Tatham NE, Wilson WH, Iranmanesh A, et al. Pathophysiology of hypercortisolism in depression. *Acta Psychiatr Scand Suppl.* 2007; (433): 90–103.

58 Belmaker RH, Agam G. Major depressive disorder. *N Engl J Med.* 2008; 358(1): 55–68.

59 Louis C, Cohen C, Depoortère R, Griebel G. Antidepressant-like effects of the corticotropin-releasing factor 1 receptor antagonist, SSR125543, and the vasopressin 1b receptor antagonist, SSR149415, in a DRL-72 s schedule in the rat. *Neuropsychopharmacology.* 2006; 31(10): 2180–7.

60 Fadgyas-Stanculete M, Buga A-M, Popa-Wagner A, Dumitrascu DL. The relationship between irritable bowel syndrome and psychiatric disorders: from molecular changes to clinical manifestations. *J Mol Psychiatry.* 2014; 2 (1): 4.

61 Farzi A, Fröhlich EE. Holzer P. Gut microbiota and the neuroendocrine system. *Neurotherapeutics.* 2018; 15(1): 5–22.

62 Dinan TG, Cryan JF. The microbiome–gut–brain axis in health and disease. *Gastroenterol Clin North Am.* 2017; 46(1): 77–89.

63 Frank MG, Thompson BM, Watkins LR, Maier SF. Glucocorticoids mediate stress-induced priming of microglial pro-inflammatory responses. *Brain Behav Immun.* 2012; 26(2): 337–45.

64 Westfall S, Pasinetti GM. The gut microbiota links dietary polyphenols with management of psychiatric mood disorders. *Front Neurosci.* 2019; 13: 1196.

65 Bancos I, Schorr Haines M, Wexler J. Adrenal fatigue, 2020. Available from: www.hormone.org/diseases-and-conditions/adrenal-fatigue

66 Cadegiani FA, Kater CE. Adrenal fatigue does not exist: a systematic review. *BMC Endocr Disord.* 2016; 16(1): 48.

Chapter

Disorders of the Thyroid and Parathyroid

Aoife M. Egan and Diana S. Dean

Background: Thyroid Hormone Synthesis and Action

The thyroid gland is located anteriorly at the base of the neck and typically weighs 10–20 g in healthy adults (1). The thyroid primarily secretes two hormones: thyroxine (T4) and triiodothyronine (T3). Their production involves a complex process including the uptake of iodide by active transport, biosynthesis and oxidation of iodide to thyroglobulin and oxidative coupling of two iodotyrosines into iodothyronines (2). T4 is produced in the thyroid gland only, but T3 is produced in both the thyroid gland and peripheral tissues by deiodination of T4. T3 occupies the nuclear receptors that mediate most of the physiological actions of thyroid hormones (3). As outlined in Figure 6.1, the hypothalamus produces thyrotropin-releasing hormone (TRH), which stimulates thyroid-stimulating hormone (TSH) production in the anterior pituitary. TSH in turn stimulates the production and release of T4 and T3 from the thyroid gland. A negative feedback loop controls this system.

Thyroid hormones are critical for brain and somatic development in infants, and in adults they affect the functioning of virtually every organ system by altering rates of protein synthesis and substrate turnover (4). Approximately 70–80% of the total body pool of thyroid hormone receptors are distributed in the adult brain (5), and there is a significant body of evidence supporting the hypothesis that thyroid hormones have a modulating impact on the brain serotonin system (6). The serotonin system plays a key role in the pathogenesis of mood disorders and forms a target for current antidepressant therapies (7). Therefore, it is not surprising that thyroid dysfunction is associated with mental health disorders. Abnormalities of thyroid function may be broadly categorised as hypothyroidism or thyrotoxicosis, and common aetiologies are outlined in Table 6.1.

Thyroid Function and Mood: Epidemiological Studies

Epidemiological studies evaluating the association between thyroid function and mood are heterogeneous in design and report varying results. The larger studies demonstrate no effect or an increase in depression with decreasing TSH concentrations (7). For example, Engum et al. assessed 30,589 individuals aged 40–89 years. They found no statistical association between thyroid dysfunction and self-rating of depression and anxiety as measured by the Hospital Anxiety and Depression Scale (HADS) (8). A prospective cohort study of 2,269 men aged 45–59 years explored whether there was an association between thyroid function in the normal range and minor psychiatric morbidity. The authors found a positive association between levels of total T4 and chronic psychiatric morbidity, but this was not persistent after adjustment for variables including social class, alcohol and smoking

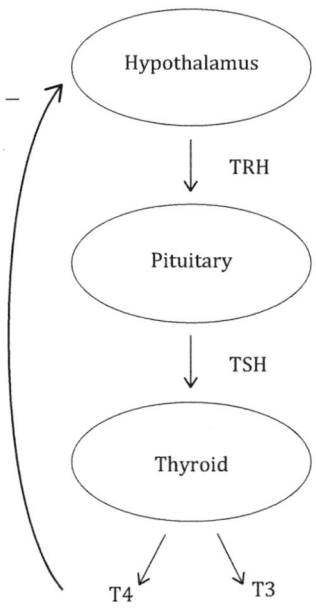

Figure 6.1 The hypothalamic–pituitary–thyroid axis. T3: triiodothyronine; T4: thyroxine; TRH: thyroid-releasing hormone; TSH: thyroid-stimulating hormone.

behaviours (9). However, the authors then undertook a systematic review and meta-analysis of six studies (including the aforementioned study) and found that there was a positive association between depression and T4 and an inverse association between depression and TSH (9).

These data point towards thyrotoxicosis rather than hypothyroidism as being associated with mood disorders. However, when interpreting these results, one must bear in mind that in community-based studies individuals with severe thyroid dysfunction will be lower in prevalence compared to those with milder disease, and therefore certain associations may be missed. This is exemplified by a study in Brazil that identified only those with more severe hypothyroidism (TSH > 10 mIU/L) (10). Here, the authors examined 1,298 middle-aged women and found that higher levels of TSH were associated with an increased risk of developing depression. Patient selection may therefore explain some of the discrepancy between these population-based studies and clinical experience.

Thyrotoxicosis

Thyrotoxicosis is the clinical manifestation of excess thyroid hormone action at the tissue level due to inappropriately high circulating thyroid hormone concentrations (11). The majority of patients with overt thyrotoxicosis will display symptoms reflective of their hypermetabolic state, including tension, hyperactivity or autonomic disturbance. Concentration is typically impaired, with restlessness, irritability and rapid thoughts and speech. Sleep disturbance is common (12). Some individuals will develop an overt psychiatric disorder such as anxiety, hypomania or mania (13). However, older individuals in particular may present with 'apathetic thyrotoxicosis', including symptoms of weakness and lethargy leading to an incorrect diagnosis of depression (14).

Table 6.1 Causes of thyroid dysfunction.[a]

Hypothyroidism
Autoimmune hypothyroidism (Hashimoto's thyroiditis)
Iatrogenic (e.g. post-thyroidectomy, radioactive iodine therapy, neck irradiation)
Iodine deficiency
Congenital hypothyroidism
Drug induced
Pituitary dysfunction
Thyroiditis

Thyrotoxicosis
Graves' disease
Toxic multinodular goitre
Solitary toxic nodule
Thyroiditis (e.g. de Quervain's, post-partum, lymphocytic)
Medication induced (e.g. excessive thyroid hormone, amiodarone)
Iodine excess
Struma ovarii
Metastatic follicular thyroid cancer
Secondary hyperthyroidism (e.g. TSH-secreting pituitary adenoma)
HCG mediated (hyperemesis gravidarum, trophoblastic disease)

[a] Not an exhaustive list.
HCG: human chorionic gonadotrophin; TSH: thyroid-stimulating hormone.

Graves' disease, an autoimmune syndrome characterised by hyperthyroidism with circulating TSH receptor antibodies, is one of the most common causes of thyrotoxicosis (15). When Robert Graves described the disease in 1835, he specifically mentioned the associated neurosis (16). Since that time, multiple studies have described the association of all aetiologies of overt thyrotoxicosis and various mood disorders (17). Hu et al. examined patients who were diagnosed with hyperthyroidism between 2000 and 2010 in the Taiwan National Health Insurance Database. This cohort consisted of 21,574 patients and the comparison cohort consisted of 21,574 matched control patients without hyperthyroidism. The incidence of bipolar disorders (incidence rate ratio = 2.31, 95% confidence interval (CI) = 1.80–2.99, $p < 0.001$) was higher for the hyperthyroidism patients than the control patients (18). A case–control study including 36 patients with newly diagnosed Graves' disease and 30 age- and sex-matched controls found that the frequency of generalised anxiety disorder was more significant in the Graves' disease group. Fourteen of the Graves' disease patients received both anti-thyroid and anti-psychotropic medications and the remainder received anti-thyroid medications only, with no difference in outcomes between the two groups (19). Finally, a Danish register-based national cohort study noted that prior to the diagnosis of hyperthyroidism, individuals had an increased risk of being hospitalised with psychiatric diagnoses (odds ratio (OR) = 1.33, 95% CI = 0.98–1.80) and an increased risk of being treated with psychotropic medications, including antipsychotics, antidepressants or anxiolytics (20).

Subclinical hyperthyroidism is a milder form of thyroid dysfunction and is defined biochemically as low or undetectable TSH and normal levels of T4 and T3 levels (21). Thus far, observational studies do not support an association between subclinical hyperthyroidism and mood disorders (17).

Hypothyroidism

Hypothyroidism may be described as the clinical manifestation of inadequate thyroid hormone action at the tissue level due to inappropriately low circulating thyroid hormone concentrations. The initial behavioural and psychological changes in adult primary hypothyroidism are not specific but usually consist of difficulties with attention, ability to concentrate, understanding complex questions and memory. With worsening of the hypothyroid state, the patient can become progressively drowsy and ultimately lapse into a coma (12). Early descriptions of myxoedema, a term used to describe severe hypothyroidism, detailed the associated psychotic changes termed 'myxoedema madness'. Specific presentations included delusions, hallucinations and acute and chronic mania (22). More recently, in 2005, Wu et al. identified a higher prevalence of hypothyroidism in patients with a major depressive disorder compared with the general population in Taiwan (1.20% versus 0.30%, OR = 3.08, 95% CI = 2.35–4.03) (23). Although limited by study size, Gulseren et al. found that anxiety and depressive symptoms as measured by the Hamilton Anxiety Rating Scale (HARS) and Hamilton Depression Rating Scale (HDRS) were more severe in patients with overt hypothyroidism (n = 33) compared to healthy controls (n = 20) (24). In addition, case series have described primary hypothyroidism presenting with acute mania as showing clinical improvement following thyroid hormone replacement therapy and psychotropic medication (17, 25). Subclinical hypothyroidism is defined based on laboratory tests identifying an elevated TSH concentration but a normal thyroid hormone concentration (21). Conflicting data are available on the association between subclinical hypothyroidism and mental health disorders. For example, a cross-sectional study based in central England identified 168 elderly subjects with subclinical hypothyroidism and found no independent association between TSH levels and depression or anxiety as measured by the HADS (26). On the other hand, a Brazil-based study (also undertaken in an elderly population) found that subclinical hypothyroidism increased the risk of depression by over fourfold (OR = 4.89; 95% CI = 2.77–8.63), and the effect was greater than that seen with overt hypothyroidism. The diagnosis of depression was based on the Structured Clinical Interview of the *Diagnostic and Statistical Manual of Mental Disorders*, 4th edition (DSM-IV) for mood disturbances (27).

Effects of Psychiatric Illness on Thyroid Function

The prior discussion has focused on the effects of a primary disorder of thyroid function on mental health. However, there is a body of evidence supporting the fact that thyroid function in psychiatric patients may be affected by the mental disorder itself, as well as by medications used to treat that illness (28).

Roca et al. examined thyroid function in 45 acutely hospitalised patients with major psychiatric disorders and found that 22 (49%) had significant elevations in thyroid hormone levels (two or more standard deviations above the mean value of controls), correlating with the severity of psychiatric symptomatology. This was accompanied by an elevation in TSH, suggesting a centrally mediated process (29). A more recent study including 81 psychotic patients with no history of thyroid dysfunction found that, compared with controls, these patients had higher free T4 concentrations, especially in the absence of prior antipsychotic therapy (30). Further examination of 86 adult acutely psychotic patients admitted to a psychiatric facility found that antipsychotic drug treatment was associated with an overall decrease in mean free T4 concentrations. However, the authors also noted that within the population there was a subgroup who experienced an increase in their low free T4 levels, suggesting a regression towards the mean (28). It is not clear whether the patients had any clinical signs of thyrotoxicosis specifically, although this would be challenging to assess in the setting of acute psychosis. This study is also limited by a lack of a control group, and so it is not clear whether changes in thyroid function are caused by treatment with antipsychotics or by remission of the psychosis. However, antipsychotics that block the action of dopamine could theoretically lead to enhanced TSH secretion by removing the inhibitory effect of dopamine on pituitary TSH secretion (28).

One must also bear in mind the entity of 'euthyroid sick syndrome', which is used to describe the disturbances in thyroid function frequently observed in seriously ill patients. This may be relevant to patients with severe psychosis or those who develop psychotic symptoms in the setting of an intercurrent illness. The typical pattern observed is a reduction in T3 levels along with normal or decreased T4 and TSH levels (31). This results from increased conversion of T4 to reverse-T3, which is biologically inactive and is possibly a protective mechanism to prevent catabolism in the setting of severe illness and macronutrient restriction.

Implications for Clinical Practice

Based on the evidence presented, thyroid dysfunction is often high on the differential diagnosis when a patient presents with a mental health disorder. Indeed, laboratory evaluation typically forms part of the baseline medical evaluation of such patients. As there is significant overlap between symptoms that may reflect an underlying thyroid disorder versus a psychiatric disorder, clinical examination is often helpful (Table 6.2). For example, if a patient with psychotic symptoms also presents with a goitre and abnormalities on eye examination, one must have a high suspicion for underlying hyperthyroidism.

Table 6.3 outlines typical biochemical findings associated with specific thyroid disorders. Speciality input may be necessary in the case of discordant thyroid function tests and to guide further workup and treatment of the underlying thyroid pathology. If the psychiatric symptoms are related to thyroid dysfunction, one should anticipate improvement with treatment of the thyroid disorder.

The Effect of Psychotropic Medications on Thyroid Function

Some psychotropic medications may have a significant effect on thyroid function, most notably lithium. Lithium is concentrated by the thyroid, inhibits iodine uptake and may inhibit thyroid hormone secretion (32). As a result, it is associated with goitre and hypothyroidism. Lithium has been associated with an increased prevalence of clinical hypothyroidism (OR = 5.78) and higher mean levels of TSH (due to higher sensitivity to TRH) compared with placebo in a meta-analysis of 385 studies (33). Where clinical hypothyroidism is present, it is frequently associated with elevated levels of anti-thyroid peroxidase antibodies (34). It is important to measure thyroid function on commencing lithium treatment and every six months thereafter (35, 36).

Phenothiazines, which are first-generation antipsychotic medications (including chlorpromazine, prochlorperazine, fluphenazine and trifluoperazine), have been

Table 6.2 Clinical features of thyroid disease.

Hypothyroidism	Thyrotoxicosis
Weight gain	Weight loss
Cold intolerance	Heat intolerance
Bradycardia	Tachycardia
Dry skin	Atrial fibrillation
Hair loss	Rapid speech
Constipation	Tremor
Slow relaxing reflexes	Diarrhoea
Menorrhagia	Proximal muscle weakness
Periorbital oedema	Hyperreflexia
Pleural and pericardial effusions	Lid retraction[a]
	Lid lag
	Exophthalmos[a]
	Palpable goitre or thyroid nodule(s)
	Thyroid bruit[a]
	Pretibial myxoedema[a]
	Thyroid acropachy
	Oligomenorrhoea/amenorrhoea

Both hypothyroidism and thyrotoxicosis are associated with a broad spectrum of behavioural and psychiatric changes outlined in the text.
[a] Features more specifically associated with Graves' disease.

Table 6.3 Typical biochemical findings associated with disorders of thyroid function.

Cause	TSH	Free T4
Primary hypothyroidism	↑	↓
Secondary hypothyroidism	↓	↓
Subclinical hypothyroidism	↑	↔
Thyrotoxicosis (primary)	↓	↑
Secondary hyperthyroidism	↑	↑
Subclinical hyperthyroidism	↓	↔
Euthyroid sick syndrome	↔/↓	↔/↓

Note: It is not uncommon for thyroid function tests to be discordant, and in this scenario a detailed history, clinical examination and review of all testing by a specialist are suggested.
T4: thyroxine; TSH: thyroid-stimulating hormone.

associated with autoimmune hypothyroidism through their effect on iodine capture and deactivation (37). Quetiapine, a second-generation antipsychotic, has been associated with suppression of thyroid function, although not with clinical hypothyroidism (38).

Tricyclic antidepressants (TCAs) also deactivate iodine and interfere with the hypothalamic–pituitary–thyroid axis by reducing the release of TSH in response to TRH. A systematic review of nearly 1,800 studies showed a small decrease in T4 associated with selective serotonin reuptake inhibitor (SSRI) treatment, although the authors commented on the poor quality of the included studies (39). Given the bidirectional relationship between mood disorders and thyroid function, but also the complex relationships among their treatments, it would be clinically appropriate to monitor thyroid function in all new presentations with depression and in all patients on TCAs, phenothiazines and perhaps quetiapine and SSRIs, in addition to lithium (36).

Thyroid Hormones as Treatment for Treatment-Resistant Depression in Unipolar and Bipolar Presentations

There is some evidence for the use of thyroid hormones as an augmentation agent for depression that has failed to respond to first-line treatments. However, the systematic reviews conducted in this area have noted the poor quality of the studies examining this treatment. One study suggested that T4 should precede lithium treatment as an augmentation for resistant depression (40). This was most widely disseminated following the STAR*D trial, which demonstrated modest benefit for the use of T3 as an adjunctive agent in resistant depression, with no significant difference from lithium (41). In a review of the use of T3 as an adjuvant treatment for resistant depression published in 2018, Parmentier and Sienaert noted that while the included studies reported improvements, their poor quality limited the extent of the conclusions that could be drawn (42). In the UK, National Institute for Health and Care Excellence (NICE) guidelines conclude that there is insufficient evidence to recommend this treatment (43). In a small randomised controlled trial (RCT), Walshaw et al. suggested that T4 might be more effective than T3 as an augmenting agent in the treatment of resistant rapid cycling bipolar disorder (44). Two RCTs of supraphysiological doses of T4 in bipolar disorder failed to find any significant improvements (45, 46). In a systematic review of the efficacy of thyroid hormones more broadly as an adjuvant treatment for resistant depression, Lorentzen et al. found that thyroid hormones were superior neither to lithium adjuvant treatment nor indeed to placebo. They concluded that there is insufficient evidence to support the use of adjunctive thyroid hormone (47). The *Maudsley Prescribing Guidelines in Psychiatry* refer to 'one failed RCT' and comments on limited efficacy in the management of bipolar disorder (36).

Background: Disorders of the Parathyroid Glands

The four parathyroid glands are typically located posteriorly to the thyroid gland and play a key role in regulating serum calcium concentrations, primarily through the secretion of parathyroid hormone (PTH). PTH, which comprises 84 amino acids, acts on the kidneys to increase calcium reabsorption and on the intestines to promote absorption of calcium, and it also stimulates increased bone turnover (48). All of these functions serve to mobilise calcium into the blood.

Disturbances in parathyroid function can result in hypercalcaemia and hypocalcaemia, and both of these scenarios are associated with the development of psychiatric symptoms. Therefore, assessment of the serum calcium concentration forms part of the baseline medical assessment of patients presenting with new psychological symptoms. The mechanism behind these specific symptoms is not clear, but it is probably due to the calcium disturbance rather than the PTH level per se. This hypothesis is supported by the fundamental role that calcium plays in neuronal physiology and brain function by governing the synthesis and secretion of neurotransmitters (49). Furthermore, studies report that psychological symptoms tend to be more closely associated with serum calcium concentrations and the rapidity of change in the calcium concentration than PTH concentrations (50, 51).

Hyperparathyroidism

Primary hyperparathyroidism is the most common cause of hypercalcaemia in outpatients and typically occurs due to a single hyper-functioning parathyroid adenoma. Multiglandular hyperplasia and parathyroid carcinoma represent rare causes (52). Secondary hyperparathyroidism typically occurs in the setting of chronic kidney disease and vitamin D or dietary calcium deficiency and is not typically associated with low serum calcium levels. Tertiary hyperparathyroidism describes excessive PTH secretion due to autonomous parathyroid function with resultant hypercalcaemia. It is rare and typically occurs after a prolonged period of secondary hyperparathyroidism with persistent parathyroid gland stimulation.

Over 50% of patients with primary hyperparathyroidism are thought to experience psychological symptoms (53). These disturbances generally consist of a lack of initiative and depression, but a number of case reports describe presentations of acute psychosis with no prior history of mental illness in the setting a of new diagnosis of primary hyperparathyroidism with hypercalcaemia (51, 54, 55). Solomon et al. evaluated psychological symptoms in 18 patients with primary hyperparathyroidism using the Symptom Checklist-90-Revised and compared them to 20 patients with benign thyroid disease. All patients were assessed before and after surgery (56). The hyperparathyroid patients showed multidimensional psychological symptom distress preoperatively in the areas of obsession–compulsion, interpersonal sensitivity, depression, anxiety, hostility and psychoticism. By one month post-operatively, the hyperparathyroid group had approached the normative mean in terms of psychological symptoms.

Reassuringly, these reports all demonstrate the reversibility of symptoms with correction of the hypercalcaemia. The links between secondary and tertiary hyperparathyroidism and psychological symptoms are not clear. However, neuropsychiatric symptoms are associated with renal dysfunction and can significantly affect disease course and quality of life in patients with chronic kidney disease (57).

Hypoparathyroidism

Hypoparathyroidism typically occurs iatrogenically after endocrine surgeries, but may also have an autoimmune aetiology with destruction of the parathyroid glands. Pesudohypoparathyroidism is a syndrome of tissue resistance to the action of PTH and is actually associated with elevated PTH levels (52). These conditions are relatively rare, and there is a paucity of studies describing the psychological associations. A review of 268 cases of hypoparathyroidism noted that 12% had neurotic symptoms, 11% had psychoses and

21% had non-specific psychiatric presentations (58, 59). It would be expected that treatment of the hypocalcaemia would lead to resolution of the symptoms. However, the clinical management of hypoparathyroidism can be challenging, and Arneiro et al. reported that a cohort of 37 patients with treated hypoparathyroidism had an increase in the number of self-reported psychological symptoms compared to a control group (60). In this study, symptom severity as measured by the Global Severity Index (GSI) was not associated with serum calcium.

Conclusion

Psychological symptoms commonly occur as a result of both thyroid and parathyroid disorders. Biochemical assessment of thyroid function and calcium concentrations should form part of the baseline assessment in those who present with new psychological symptoms. Once an abnormality is confirmed, further workup and treatment of the underlying endocrine disorder can be expected to alleviate and even reverse the psychological symptoms. It is hoped that future research will clarify the association between milder abnormalities of thyroid function and mood and further evaluate the interactions between psychiatric illness, psychotropic medications and thyroid function.

References

1   Pankow B, Michalak J, McGee MK. Adult human thyroid weight. *Health Phys.* 1985; 49(6): 1097–103.

2   Kopp P, Carlos Solis-S J. Thyroid hormone synthesis. In: *Clinical Management of Thyroid Disease* (eds. FE Wondisford, S Radowick). Elsevier, 2009, pp. 19–41.

3   Yen P. *Genomic and Nongenomic Actions of Thyroid Hormones.* Lippincott Williams & Wilkins, 2005.

4   Brent GA. Thyroid hormone action. UpToDate. Available from: www.uptodate.com/contents/thyroid-hormone-action?search=thyroidmenta&source=search_result&selectedTitle=3~150&usage_type=default&display_rank=3 - H1. Published 2018

5   Fukao A, Takamatsu J, Arishima T, Tanaka M, Kawai T, Okamoto Y, et al. Graves' disease and mental disorders. *J Clin Transl Endocrinol.* 2020; 19: 100207.

6   Bauer M, Heinz A, Whybrow PC. Thyroid hormones, serotonin and mood: of synergy and significance in the adult brain. *Mol Psychiatry.* 2002; 7(2): 140–56.

7   Dayan CM, Panicker V. Hypothyroidism and depression. *Eur Thyroid J.* 2013; 2(3): 168–79.

8   Engum A, Bjøro T, Mykletun A, Dahl AA. An association between depression, anxiety and thyroid function – a clinical fact or an artefact? *Acta Psychiatr Scand.* 2002; 106 (1): 27–34.

9   Williams MD, Harris R, Dayan CM, Evans J, Gallacher J, Ben-Shlomo Y. Thyroid function and the natural history of depression: findings from the Caerphilly Prospective Study (CaPS) and a meta-analysis. *Clin Endocrinol (Oxf).* 2009; 70 (3): 484–92.

10 Guimarães JM, de Souza Lopes C, Baima J, Sichieri R. Depression symptoms and hypothyroidism in a population-based study of middle-aged Brazilian women. *J Affect Disord.* 2009; 117(1–2): 120–3.

11 Sharma A, Stan MN. Thyrotoxicosis: diagnosis and management. *Mayo Clin Proc.* 2019; 94(6): 1048–64.

12 Braverman L, Utiger R. *Werner and Ingbar's The Thyroid,* 6th ed. J.B. Lippincott Company, 1991.

13 Bunevicius R, Prange AJ. Thyroid disease and mental disorders: cause and effect or only comorbidity? *Curr Opin Psychiatry.* 2010; 23(4): 363–8.

14 Wu W, Sun Z, Yu J, Meng Q, Wang M, Miao J, Sun L. A clinical retrospective

analysis of factors associated with apathetic hyperthyroidism. *Pathobiology.* 2010; 77 (1): 46–51.

15 McLachlan S, Pegg C, Atherton M, Middleton S, Clark F, Rees Smith B. TSH receptor antibody synthesis by thyroid lymphocytes. *Clin Endocrinol (Oxf).* 1986; 24(2): 223–30.

16 Graves R. Newly observed affection of the thyroid gland in females. *Lond Med Surg J.* 1835; 7: 516–7.

17 Ritchie M, Yeap BB. Thyroid hormone: influences on mood and cognition in adults. *Maturitas.* 2015; 81(2): 266–75.

18 Hu L-Y, Shen C-C, Hu Y-W, Chen M-H, Tsai C-F, Chiang H-L, et al. Hyperthyroidism and risk for bipolar disorders: a nationwide population-based study. *PLoS ONE.* 2013; 8(8): e73057.

19 Chattopadhyay C, Chakrabarti N, Ghosh S. An assessment of psychiatric disturbances in Graves disease in a medical college in eastern India. *Niger J Clin Pract.* 2012; 15 (3): 276–9.

20 Brandt F, Thvilum M, Almind D, Christensen K, Green A, Hegedüs L, Brix TH. Hyperthyroidism and psychiatric morbidity: evidence from a Danish nationwide register study. *Eur J Endocrinol.* 2014; 170(2): 341–8.

21 Cooper DS, Biondi B. Subclinical thyroid disease. *Lancet.* 2012; 379(9821): 1142–54.

22 Asher R. Myxoedematous madness. *Br Med J.* 1949; 2(4627): 555–62.

23 Wu EL, Chien IC, Lin CH, Chou YJ, Chou P. Increased risk of hypothyroidism and hyperthyroidism in patients with major depressive disorder: a population-based study. *J Psychosom Res.* 2013; 74(3): 233–7.

24 Gulseren S, Gulseren L, Hekimsoy Z, Cetinay P, Ozen C, Tokatlioglu B. Depression, anxiety, health-related quality of life, and disability in patients with overt and subclinical thyroid dysfunction. *Arch Med Res.* 2006; 37(1): 133–9.

25 Khemka D, Ali JA, Koch CA. Primary hypothyroidism associated with acute mania: case series and literature review. *Exp Clin Endocrinol Diabetes.* 2011; 119(8): 513–7.

26 Roberts LM, Pattison H, Roalfe A, Franklyn J, Wilson S, Hobbs FDR, Parle JV. Is subclinical thyroid dysfunction in the elderly associated with depression or cognitive dysfunction? *Ann Intern Med.* 2006; 145(8): 573–81.

27 Chueire VB, Romaldini JH, Ward LS. Subclinical hypothyroidism increases the risk for depression in the elderly. *Arch Gerontol Geriatr.* 2007; 44(1): 21–8.

28 Bunevicius R, Steibliene V, Prange AJ. Thyroid axis function after in-patient treatment of acute psychosis with antipsychotics: a naturalistic study. *BMC Psychiatry.* 2014; 14: 279.

29 Roca RP, Blackman MR, Ackerley MB, Harman SM, Gregerman RI. Thyroid hormone elevations during acute psychiatric illness: relationship to severity and distinction from hyperthyroidism. *Endocr Res.* 1990; 16(4): 415–47.

30 Steiblienė V, Mickuvienė N, Prange AJ, Bunevičius R. Concentrations of thyroid axis hormones in psychotic patients on hospital admission: the effects of prior drug use. *Medicina (Kaunas).* 2012; 48(5): 229–34.

31 Fliers E, Bianco AC, Langouche L, Boelen A. Thyroid function in critically ill patients. *Lancet Diabetes Endocrinol.* 2015; 3(10): 816–25.

32 Lazarus JH. The effects of lithium therapy on thyroid and thyrotropin-releasing hormone. *Thyroid.* 1998; 8(10): 909–13.

33 McKnight RF, Adida M, Budge K, Stockton S, Goodwin GM, Geddes JR. Lithium toxicity profile: a systematic review and meta-analysis. *Lancet.* 2012; 379(9817): 721–8.

34 Sauvage MF, Marquet P, Rousseau A, Raby C, Buxeraud J, Lachatre G. Relationship between psychotropic drugs and thyroid function: a review. *Toxicol Appl Pharmacol.* 1998; 149(2): 127–35.

35 Nikolova VL, Pattanaseri K, Hidalgo-Mazzei D, Taylor D, Young AH. Is lithium monitoring NICE? Lithium monitoring in a UK secondary care setting. *J Psychopharmacol.* 2018; 32(4): 408–15.

36 Taylor DM, Paton C, Kapur S. *The Maudsley Prescribing Guidelines in Psychiatry*, 12th ed. Wiley Blackwell, 2015.

37 Bou Khalil R, Richa S. Thyroid adverse effects of psychotropic drugs: a review. *Clin Neuropharmacol*. 2011; 34(6): 248–55.

38 Li C, Lai J, Huang T, Han Y, Du Y, Xu Y, Hu S. Thyroid functions in patients with bipolar disorder and the impact of quetiapine monotherapy: a retrospective, naturalistic study. *Neuropsychiatr Dis Treat*. 2019; 15: 2285–90.

39 Caye A, Pilz LK, Maia AL, Hidalgo MP, Furukawa TA, Kieling C. The impact of selective serotonin reuptake inhibitors on the thyroid function among patients with major depressive disorder: a systematic review and meta-analysis. *Eur Neuropsychopharmacol*. 2020; 33: 139–45.

40 Spoov J, Lahdelma L. Should thyroid augmentation precede lithium augmentation – a pilot study. *J Affect Disord*. 1998; 49(3): 235–9.

41 Nierenberg AA, Fava M, Trivedi MH, Wisniewski SR, Thase ME, McGrath PJ, et al. A comparison of lithium and T(3) augmentation following two failed medication treatments for depression: a STAR*D report. *Am J Psychiatry*. 2006; 163 (9): 1519–30; quiz 1665.

42 Parmentier T, Sienaert P. The use of triiodothyronine (T3) in the treatment of bipolar depression: a review of the literature. *J Affect Disord*. 2018; 229: 410–4.

43 National Institute for Health and Care Excellence. Depression in Adults: Recognition and Management (Clinical Guideline 90), 2009. Available from: www .nice.org.uk/guidance/cg90

44 Walshaw PD, Gyulai L, Bauer M, Bauer MS, Calimlim B, Sugar CA, Whybrow PC. Adjunctive thyroid hormone treatment in rapid cycling bipolar disorder: a double-blind placebo-controlled trial of levothyroxine (L-T_4) and triiodothyronine (T_3). *Bipolar Disord*. 2018; 20(7): 594–603.

45 Pilhatsch M, J Stamm T, Stahl P, Lewitzka U, Berghöfer A, Sauer C, et al. Treatment of bipolar depression with supraphysiologic doses of levothyroxine: a randomized, placebo-controlled study of comorbid anxiety symptoms. *Int J Bipolar Disord*. 2019; 7(1): 21.

46 Stamm TJ, Lewitzka U, Sauer C, Pilhatsch M, Smolka MN, Koeberle U, et al. Supraphysiologic doses of levothyroxine as adjunctive therapy in bipolar depression: a randomized, double-blind, placebo-controlled study. *J Clin Psychiatry*. 2014; 75 (2): 162–8.

47 Lorentzen R, Nørgaard Kjaer J, Dinesen Østergaard S, Madsen MM. Thyroid hormone treatment in the management of treatment-resistant unipolar depression: a systematic review and meta-analysis. *Acta Psychiatr Scand*. 2020; 141(4): 316–26.

48 Marx SJ. Hyperparathyroid and hypoparathyroid disorders. *N Engl J Med*. 2000; 343(25): 1863–75.

49 Rajagopal S, Ponnusamy M. Calcium signalling in neurological disorders. In: *Calcium Signaling: From Physiology to Diseases* (eds. S Rajagopal, M Ponnusamy). Springer, 2017, pp. 43–60.

50 Park S, Hieber R. Acute psychosis secondary to suspected hyperparathyroidism: a case report and literature review. *Ment Health Clin*. 2016; 6 (6): 304–7.

51 Alarcón RD, Franceschini JA. Hyperparathyroidism and paranoid psychosis. Case report and review of the literature. *Br J Psychiatry*. 1984; 145: 477–86.

52 Michels TC, Kelly KM. Parathyroid disorders. *Am Fam Physician*. 2013; 88(4): 249–57.

53 Petersen P. Psychiatric disorders in primary hyperparathyroidism. *J Clin Endocrinol Metab*. 1968; 28(10): 1491–5.

54 Papa A, Bononi F, Sciubba S, Ursella S, Gentiloni-Silveri N. Primary hyperparathyroidism: acute paranoid psychosis. *Am J Emerg Med*. 2003; 21(3): 250–1.

55 Babar G, Alemzadeh R. A case of acute psychosis in an adolescent male. *Case Rep Endocrinol*. 2014; 2014: 937631.

56 Solomon BL, Schaaf M, Smallridge RC. Psychologic symptoms before and after parathyroid surgery. *Am J Med*. 1994; 96 (2): 101–6.

57 Szeifert L, Adorjáni G, Zalai D, Novák M. [Mood disorders in patients with chronic kidney disease: significance, etiology and prevalence of depression]. *Orv Hetil*. 2009; 150(13): 589–96.

58 Velasco PJ, Manshadi M, Breen K, Lippmann S. Psychiatric aspects of parathyroid disease. *Psychosomatics*. 1999; 40(6): 486–90.

59 Denko JD, Kaelbling R. The psychiatric aspects of hypoparathyroidism. *Acta Psychiatr Scand Suppl*. 1962; 38(164): 1–70.

60 Arneiro AJ, Duarte BCC, Kulchetscki RM, Cury VBS, Lopes MP, Kliemann BS, et al. Self-report of psychological symptoms in hypoparathyroidism patients on conventional therapy. *Arch Endocrinol Metab*. 2018; 62(3): 319–24.

Psychological Factors Impacting on Endocrine Disorders and Self-Management and Medication-Taking Behaviour

Eimear Morrissey, Seán F. Dinneen and Anne M. Doherty

Self-management and medication-taking behaviour including lifestyle change is essential for the stabilisation of any endocrine condition; however, many patients struggle to achieve this. This chapter will address underlying reasons for this and discuss psychological approaches to optimising self-management and medication-taking behaviour.

The majority of endocrine conditions can be successfully managed with long-term treatment, whether that be in the form of medication or lifestyle factors. In order for treatment to be effective, self-management and medication-taking behaviour is key. The World Health Organization (WHO) defines adherence to long-term therapy as 'the extent to which a person's behaviour – taking medication, following a diet and/or executing lifestyle changes – corresponds with agreed recommendations from a health care provider' (1). Central to the concept of adherence or self-management and medication-taking behaviour is the presumption of an agreement between prescriber and patient about the prescriber's recommendations – and for treatment or self-management to be effective, it is important to have a genuine agreement.

Difficulties with self-management and medication-taking behaviour occur when a patient does not initiate a new prescription, implement it as prescribed or persist with treatment (2). The WHO has posited that, in general, there are five dimensions to self-management and medication-taking behaviour, and all of them can impact on rates of difficulties with self-management: condition-related factors; health system factors; socio-economic factors; therapy-related factors; and patient-related factors (1). While these dimensions are not entirely independent of each other, this serves as a useful means for organising the broad range of factors that can contribute to difficulties with self-management.

Maintaining self-management and medication-taking behaviour can be challenging, particularly for those living with long-term or comorbid physical and mental health conditions.

Take, for example, difficulties with self-management of treatment in type 2 diabetes, which can be costly, both to the individual and to the healthcare system. Medication for type 2 diabetes has proven efficacy if taken as recommended (3, 4). However, if less than 80% of the prescribed medication is taken, only half the expected reduction in blood glucose control is seen, increasing the risk of complications for this population (5). Despite this, ideal medication-taking behaviour is suboptimal for at least half the population of people with type 2 diabetes prescribed these medications (6). This suboptimal rate of medication-taking behaviour leads to higher HbA1c values, significantly increased morbidity and mortality, increased use of healthcare resources, increased hospitalisations and higher medical costs (6). The cost of difficulties with self-management and diabetes medication-taking behaviour in the UK has been estimated at £100 million per year in avoidable treatment costs (7).

Much research has been done into the barriers to self-management and medication-taking behaviour in those living with type 2 diabetes. A recent systematic review examined 196 studies on the topic and found that the common barriers reported included regimen complexity (medication-taking behaviour decreased when more than two medications were used daily), side effects of medication, memory problems, depression, environmental factors (e.g. cost and access to medication) and patients' beliefs regarding the benefit of treatment (8). The link between depression and difficulties with self-management and medication-taking behaviour in type 2 diabetes is a well-established one. A 2008 meta-analysis pooled 47 studies (over 17,000 participants) and found the association between depression and difficulties with self-management and medication-taking behaviour in diabetes to be significant, with a moderate effect size (9). A later meta-analysis found that people living with depression were 1.76-times more likely to have difficulties with medication-taking behaviour for chronic disease than people without depression and that this association was similar across all chronic conditions (10).

As depression is twice as common in people living with type 2 diabetes than the general population, this relationship is one that warrants examination (11). It is possible that as the physical and psychological needs of diabetes and depression compete with each other, under-regulation, where the characteristics of one condition conflict with the management of the other, may occur (12). This is discussed in more detail in Chapter 2. Motivation is a key factor in the initiation and maintenance of self-management and medication-taking behaviour, and the reduction in motivation that is commonly seen in depression may interfere with this process.

Addiction and Barriers to Self-Management

Addictions may present significant difficulties for the self-management of chronic diseases. When someone has an addiction, this tends to be their priority, often to the exclusion of other things in the person's life. It is difficult to prioritise self-management of diabetes or any other condition while the addiction is in the foreground, regardless of what that addiction is to (alcohol, drugs, gambling, etc.). In addition, alcohol is depressogenic, and as such may impede self-management due to suboptimal mood.

In the case of alcohol, there are a number of specific issues from a diabetes point of view. Alcohol excess may increase the risk of developing type 2 diabetes (13), although light or moderate alcohol intake may be protective against atherosclerotic disorders (14).

Harmful use of alcohol is associated with increased risk of pancreatitis, which, when chronic, is associated with an increased risk of diabetes: approximately 40% of cases may result in diabetes mellitus, some requiring insulin (15). Diabetic neuropathy can be exacerbated by the neuropathy secondary to alcohol misuse and vitamin B_{12} deficiency (16). Chronic heavy alcohol use is also associated with hypertension and an elevated risk of cardiovascular events (17).

In people with diabetes, alcohol (when being metabolised by the liver) inhibits gluconeogenesis, and as a result it is associated with an increased risk of hypoglycaemia.

When combined with a carbohydrate-heavy meal or where the alcohol itself has a high sugar content (e.g. cocktails, high-sugar mixers and ciders), ingestion of alcohol may result in significant fluctuations in blood glucose, contribute to risk of hyperglycaemia and hypoglycaemia and affect the proportion of time spent in the target blood glucose range (18).

Psychological Models Underlying Difficulties with Self-Management and Medication-Taking Behaviour

Psychological theories of health behaviour and health behaviour change have been developed in order to understand and explain the difficulties with self-management and medication-taking behaviour across many conditions. When considering self-management, the difference between intentional and unintentional difficulties with self-management and medication-taking behaviour need to be considered. Intentional or conscious difficulties with self-management and medication-taking behaviour refer to a situation in which the patient chooses to deviate from the agreed treatment plan. Unintentional difficulties with self-management and medication-taking behaviour are more passive processes in which the patient may be forgetful or careless with regards to treatment or may not be able to access the prescribed treatment.

Reflective–Impulsive Model

Strack and Deutsch's reflective–impulsive model is a dual-process model in which they propose that our behaviours are driven by two systems (19). The first is the reflective process, which is the effortful process through which the individual is consciously aware and in control, carrying out the behaviour based on conscious deliberation. The second process is the impulsive process; this requires little cognitive capacity and operates quickly and automatically, requiring minimal effort, and it is the default process in determining behaviour. Given this default role, the impulsive process drives behaviour unless there is a capacity and need for conscious decision-making.

Common Sense Model of Self-Regulation

Intentional or conscious difficulties with self-management and medication-taking behaviour tend to take place within the reflective system, as the person actively decides not to engage with their treatment. The common sense model of self-regulation (CSM-SR) provides a useful model to understand reflection and motivation (20). The CSM-SR incorporates elements of other health behaviour theories and has been used in several illness contexts (including diabetes) to predict patients' self-management and medication-taking behaviour (21). It posits that an individual's illness identity, causes, timeline, consequences and control beliefs affect their behaviours in response to a health threat, including their medication-taking behaviour (22).

Control beliefs refer to the degree of control the patient believes they have over their condition and over their healthcare delivery or treatment. These control beliefs, particularly those regarding the treatment itself (i.e. belief in the necessity of and concerns regarding the treatment), have been shown to predict self-management and medication-taking behaviour (23). The necessity–concerns framework (NCF) suggests that a relationship exists between two separate dimensions (the patient's necessity beliefs and their concerns regarding

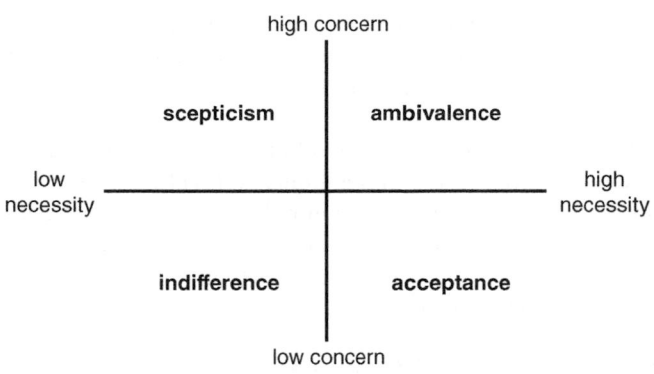

Figure 7.1 The necessity–concerns framework (23).

medication) and between these two predictors and self-management (Figure 7.1). The NCF states that patients implicitly weigh the costs against the benefits of taking a medication when deciding whether or not to adhere to it and that medication-taking behaviours will be greater the more patients' beliefs in the necessity of the medication exceed their concerns (23).

The Beliefs about Medication Questionnaire (BMQ) was developed to assess necessity and concern beliefs. A meta-analysis of 94 publications using the BMQ by Horne et al. showed that the Specific Necessity Beliefs measure was positively and consistently related to self-management and medication-taking behaviour and Specific Concerns scores were consistently and negatively related to self-management and medication-taking behaviour (24). However, work by Verplanken has suggested that these treatment beliefs may be more predictive in the short term than in the long term, implying that they may play a larger role in the initiation rather than the maintenance of self-management and medication-taking behaviour (25). Evidence shows that treatment beliefs are associated with intentional suboptimal self-management and medication-taking behaviour, as these beliefs can represent a reflective choice on how to behave (26, 27). A good example of the NCF in action is in the case of insulin in a person living with diabulimia: in this situation, the person's concern about weight gain outweighs the perceived necessity of the insulin to maintain their blood glucose levels. This then leads to insulin omission. Further detail on eating disorders and disordered eating in diabetes is provided in Chapter 4.

Habits

Problems with unintentional difficulties with self-management and medication-taking behaviour tend to reside in the impulsive process of the dual-process model, as motivation is less of a contributing factor and the person may just be forgetting to engage with their treatment. The impulsive system is largely governed by habits – a specific form of cue–response association formed in memory as a consequence of repeated performance of a particular action in response to a particular cue context (28). Once a behaviour is more strongly influenced by the impulsive system and becomes habitual, it does not require reflection or deliberation on reasons, because habits are automatically triggered by conditioned contextual cues; for example, a person may take their medication (i.e. the behavioural response) in the morning and evening after the cue of brushing their teeth (29). A study by Phillips et al. found that habit strength predicted self-reported good self-management and medication-taking behaviour (both medication and exercise) in type 2 diabetes (30). Another recent cross-sectional study observed that the relationship between depression and difficulties with medication-taking behaviour was worse when habit strength was weak (31).

It is worth noting that the distinction between intentional suboptimal medication-taking behaviour falling in the reflective system and unintentional difficulties with self-management and medication-taking behaviour falling in the impulsive system is not totally binary (e.g. a person who is not motivated to take their medication may be more inclined to forget it). However, it serves as a useful starting point when working with a person to untangle the barriers to treatment and create a plan of support.

Difficulties with Self-Management and Medication-Taking Behaviour in the Endocrine Clinic

Identifying Barriers to Self-Management

Difficulties with self-management can sometimes be challenging to identify. Self-report measures exist, such as the Morisky Medication Adherence Scale (32). Condition-specific scales such as the Adherence in Diabetes Questionnaire and the Summary of Diabetes Self-Care Activities Measure are also available (33, 34). Other methods can also be used, such as urine or blood bioassays, checking pharmacy refill records or counting remaining pills at the end of a prescription. However, patients can often be hesitant to report difficulties with self-management and medication-taking behaviour or to express concerns about prescribed medications because of a fear that this will displease the prescriber, and screening for these difficulties may serve to worsen this perception. It is key to remember that assessing difficulties with self-management is not about monitoring patients, but rather about identifying needs for information and support (35).

Often there may be red flags that indicate a problem with intentional and/or unintentional difficulties with self-management and medication-taking behaviour. These may include worsening of symptoms or markers (e.g. an unusually high HbA1c value) or repeated missed appointments or recurrent admissions with unexplained episodes of diabetic ketoacidosis (36, 37). In diabetes, where the treatment regimen may be complex, the presence of multiple comorbidities and particularly a diagnosis of depression are also predictors of difficulties with self-management and medication-taking behaviour. The person may show a lack of understanding or express doubts about the treatment regimen. In the case of these red flags, the first step to facilitating improved self-management and medication-taking behaviour is to take a 'no-blame approach' and encourage an open and honest conversation to identify barriers to self-management and any underlying drivers (29).

Sometimes the barriers to optimal self-management behaviour may be due to specific psychological problems that may arise around treatment. In diabetes, it may be worth considering whether the person has developed a needle phobia, resulting in difficulty administering insulin or GLP-1 agonists (38), or a fear of hypoglycaemia (or 'hypos') in response sometimes to unpleasant hypo experiences, which may result in the person running sugars too high in an attempt to avoid further hypos at any cost (39). Sometimes the person may be so fearful of developing the complications of diabetes that they adopt a defence mechanism of denial involving not engaging in their diabetes care, a behaviour that paradoxically raises their risk of developing complications (40). Other people may develop diabetes burnout due to the unrelenting pressure of intense self-management resulting in emotional exhaustion and frustration with self-care behaviours. Such burnout is associated with difficulties in maintaining self-management (41). Recent work in the setting of young adult type 1 diabetes clinics has highlighted the potential benefits of measuring diabetes distress as a part of routine clinical practice and in this way acknowledging the burden of living with this demanding condition (42).

Supporting Self-Management and Medication-Taking Behaviour

When addressing difficulties with self-management and medication-taking behaviour, the focus should not blindly be on getting the person to take more medication or increase their efforts at lifestyle change. Instead, it should start with a discussion of the person's thoughts on their treatment and any barriers to self-management or reasons why they are not motivated or are unable to engage with self-management. The responsibility of the health-care professional is to support people to make informed decisions about their treatment and use appropriately prescribed treatments to their best effect (35).

A useful way of understanding self-management and medication-taking behaviour in the clinic involves using the perceptions and practicalities approach (PAPA), as illustrated in Figure 7.2 (43). This approach is supported by the National Institute for Health and Care Excellence (NICE) in the UK (35). The PAPA draws on the CSM-SR and NCF and states that motivation and ability are the two key attributes to address when considering self-management and medication-taking behaviour.

Perception of treatment drives motivation for self-management and medication-taking behaviour. As outlined in the NCF, motivation is often influenced by people's beliefs around the necessity of the treatment versus their concerns with engaging with it. When exploring barriers to self-management and medication-taking behaviour with a person, it is important to help them avoid choices that are based on misconceptions and misplaced concerns, such as not taking an antidepressant tablet due to the lack of an immediate therapeutic response (44). One route of ascertaining whether a correctly informed choice has occurred is to check whether the individual can demonstrate knowledge of relevant information about the treatment (45). In the event of genuine concerns, such as unpleasant side effects, treatment recommendations should take this into account and seek to come to a shared decision on the best type of treatment possible. Tools have been developed to facilitate shared decision-making, such as the Mayo Clinic Statin Choice Decision Aid and the Mayo Clinic Diabetes Medication Decision Aid. An evolving literature in this area includes the work of Victor Montori in an area he terms 'minimally disruptive medicine', and that of Richard Lehman, who has championed the concept of a 'shared understanding of medicine'. Both approaches emphasise a patient-centred approach to care delivery and highlight the fact that the burden of illness has to be viewed in the context of the burden of self-management.

Additional traditional approaches include cognitive behavioural therapy (CBT) and motivational interviewing (MI), techniques that are helpful in challenging unhelpful beliefs and low self-efficacy and can improve perceptions of treatment (46, 47).

Practicalities of treatment drive the ability for optimal self-management and medication-taking behaviour. A common practical barrier is forgetfulness. Appropriate support can include the establishment of reminder systems and education on habit

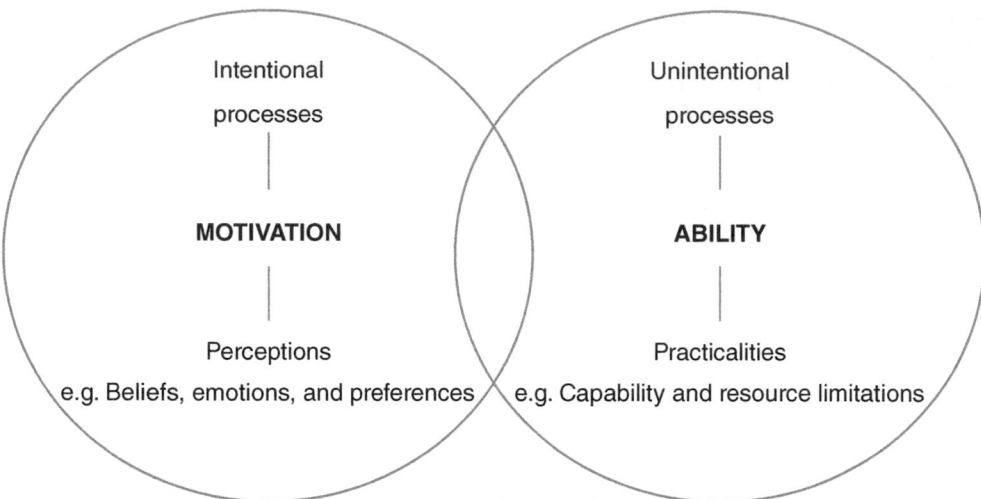

Figure 7.2 Perceptions and practicalities approach. Reproduced from (43). Reproduced with permission from *European Psychologist* 2019; 24(1): 82–96 ©2019 Hogrefe Publishing www.hogrefe.com, https://doi.org/10.1027/1016-9040/a000353

formation (i.e. linking the treatment behaviour to specific environmental cues, such as taking long-acting insulin while brushing one's teeth) (32). The complexities of the treatment regimen represent another common barrier, and simplifying the regimen and reducing unnecessary polypharmacy can aid self-management and medication-taking behaviour here. In the case of multiple medications being necessary, solutions such as fixed-dose combination tablets, blister packs and dosing boxes can be used (31). Environmental factors such as the cost of and access to treatment are more difficult barriers to tackle. A recent systematic review on diabetes medication-taking behaviour found that in the USA the type of Medicare coverage had a significant effect on medication-taking behaviour (8).

In practice, how to make use of the PAPA to address difficulties with self-management and medication-taking behaviour in the clinic can be summarised in three steps (31):

(1) Necessity beliefs: Communicate a rationale for the personal necessity of treatment that addresses the implicit question 'Why do I need to follow this treatment to achieve a goal that is important to me?' This should fit with the patient's beliefs about the illness and consider symptom expectations and experiences.
(2) Concerns: Elicit and address concerns and outstanding information needs. Provide support with side-effect management if indicated and address low self-efficacy beliefs relating to self-management and medication-taking behaviour.
(3) Practicalities: Make the treatment as easy to use as possible and support the formation of a treatment habit.

Motivational Interviewing and Cognitive Behavioural Therapy

MI is a brief therapeutic intervention that has its origins in addiction psychotherapy and that focuses on identifying the person's degree of willingness to commit to effecting change in their behaviours and exploring ambivalence towards change. The original addiction model is focused on identifying the willingness to commit to effecting personal change (46, 48, 49). In recent decades, this has moved into the area of promoting behavioural

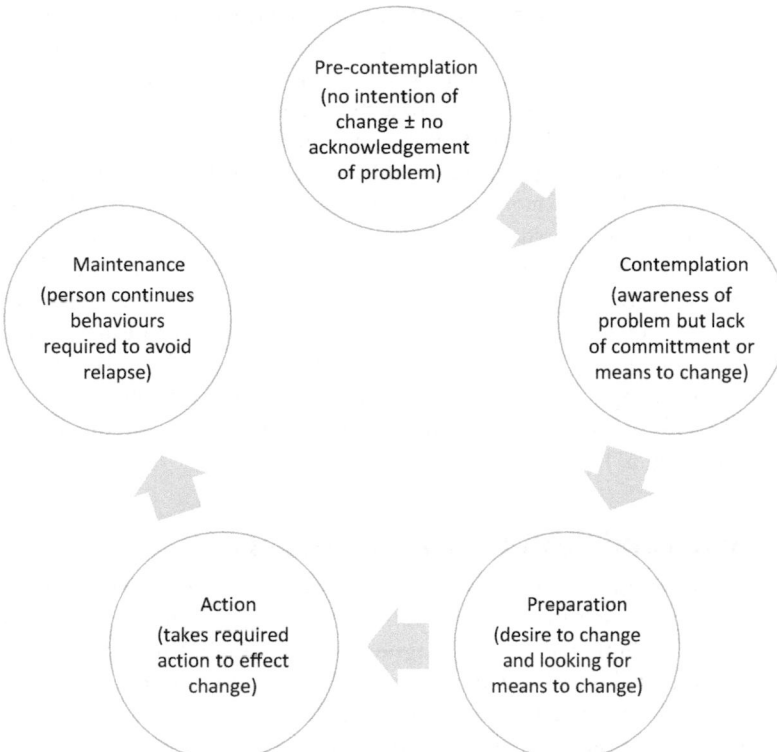

Figure 7.3 Stages of change based on the Prochaska and DiClemente (50) model.

change for reasons other than addiction, and there is a growing evidence base for its efficacy. It is based on the idea that a person may be at different stages of the 'cycle of change' (see Figure 7.3), and it considers the importance of identifying where the person is in order to inform the approach taken. It maintains a focus on moving someone along the cycle to the next stage rather than looking to achieve abstinence (or behaviour change) immediately, acknowledging that change requires time. Its ethos is of collaboration, empathy and autonomy, and it includes techniques such as expressing empathy, supporting self-efficacy, rolling with resistance, developing a sense of discrepancy between the current and the desired future, looking for 'green shoots' and asking permission to give advice (46, 50). In a systematic review, MI was associated with improved outcomes in young adults and adolescents with a range of chronic illnesses (51). There have been a number of randomised controlled trials of MI in diabetes specifically with the aim of improving self-management. Many of these showed some benefit in improving glycaemic control, such as the ADaPT and D6 studies (52, 53). Early meta-analyses suggested that MI may be associated with improvements in specific groups, but larger and more recent meta-analyses have been rather less encouraging (54–58).

There is also a growing evidence base for the use of CBT in chronic disease management. Traditional CBT was designed to treat depression and anxiety, but in recent decades it has been applied to other situations where a cycle of dysfunctional thoughts and behaviours may be challenged with benefit to the patient. This can be used in endocrinology where specific barriers to optimal self-management can be identified, such as a fear of hypoglycaemia or a disabling fear of developing the complications of diabetes that results in the person paradoxically disengaging from their diabetes care in order to avoid exposure to this anxiety. Such anxieties may be explored and challenged utilising a CBT frame – this allows any thoughts that the person might have that may be contributing to or perpetuating the anxiety to be identified and challenged using established CBT techniques. Such techniques might include keeping a diary of mood and or self-management behaviour, challenging unhelpful thoughts via Socratic questioning or behavioural experiments. For example, if a person has the thoughts that their diabetes cannot be controlled despite their best efforts and that they will end up on dialysis regardless of what they do, the therapist might explore these thoughts using Socratic questioning and perhaps asking the person to examine the evidence for their beliefs, and then perhaps moving on to using behavioural experiments to see the effect of behaviour change on blood glucose. There is evidence from systematic reviews that CBT can be effective in improving diabetes self-management in adults with type 1 and type 2 diabetes (56, 57).

Education of Patients and Healthcare Professionals

Self-management education programmes such as the Dose Adjustment for Normal Eating (DAFNE) programme for individuals living with type 1 diabetes or the Diabetes Education and Self-Management for Ongoing and Newly Diagnosed (DESMOND) programme for type 2 diabetes have become established as part of routine clinical practice in the UK and Ireland. These programmes help patients (and their significant others) gain a better understanding of their condition and, using a variety of teaching and learning methods (including vicarious or observational learning), they encourage patients to set personal goals around their self-management behaviour.

In March 2018, an All-Party Parliamentary Group (APPG) met in the British House of Commons to hear from people living with diabetes, healthcare professionals and researchers on the subject of diabetes and mental health. A report from this consultation highlighted a general lack of psychological support for people living with both type 1 and type 2 diabetes in the National Health Service (NHS). Some of the testimonies from people living with diabetes described how diabetes healthcare professionals may be more interested in discussing clinical outcomes and may feel uncomfortable or ill-equipped to discuss the psychological aspects of living with a chronic illness. The APPG report emphasised the need to make psychological services more readily available and highlighted potential benefits not just to patients, but also to diabetes specialist teams and the wider health service.

The Knuston Counselling and Empowerment Course was mentioned specifically in the APPG report as a good example of a training programme for healthcare professionals that can upskill (non-psychologist) members of primary or secondary care teams in identifying psychological issues. Based on the person-centred approach to counselling developed by Carl Rogers, the Knuston Counselling and Empowerment Course trains participants to help clients identify a specific problem, clarify the emotional aspects of that problem and come up with an action plan to try to address the issues raised during consultations. The course was originally developed in the 1980s and has evolved over the ensuing years, and it now incorporates the empowerment principles developed by Bob Anderson and Martha Funnell in Michigan. While many former participants describe it as changing their approach to delivering diabetes care, the intensive nature of the (face-to-face) course limits its potential reach and impact.

Conclusion

The majority of endocrine conditions can be successfully managed with long-term treatment, whether that be in the form of medication or lifestyle factors. In order for treatment to be effective, self-management and medication-taking behaviour is key. Self-management, including lifestyle change, is essential for the stabilisation of any endocrine condition; however, many patients struggle to achieve this. It is important to consider any underlying causes, including depression, eating disorders, addictions and diabetes-specific psychological problems (e.g. needle phobia, fear of hypoglycaemia, etc.).

The management of difficulties with self-management and medication-taking behaviour starts with identifying then addressing the underlying reasons, considering filling any educational gaps and considering psychological approaches to optimising self-management. All of this needs to be done in conjunction with the patient in a spirit of shared understanding and shared decision-making.

References

1   Sabeté E. *Adherence to Long-Term Therapies: Evidence for Action*. World Health Organization, 2003.

2   Vrijens B, Antoniou S, Burnier M, de la Sierra A, Volpe M. Current situation of medication adherence in hypertension. *Front Pharmacol*. 2017; 8: 100.

3   UK Prospective Diabetes Study Group. Efficacy of atenolol and captopril in reducing risk of macrovascular and microvascular complications in type 2 diabetes: UKPDS 39. UK Prospective Diabetes Study Group. *BMJ*. 1998; 317 (7160): 713–20.

4   Colhoun HM, Betteridge DJ, Durrington PN, Hitman GA, Neil HA, Livingstone SJ, et al. Primary prevention of cardiovascular disease with atorvastatin in type 2 diabetes in the Collaborative Atorvastatin Diabetes Study (CARDS): multicentre randomised placebo-controlled trial. *Lancet*. 2004; 364 (9435): 685–96.

5   Farmer AJ, Rodgers LR, Lonergan M, Shields B, Weedon MN, Donnelly L, et al. Adherence to oral glucose-lowering therapies and associations with 1-year HbA1c: a retrospective cohort analysis in a large primary care database. *Diabetes Care*. 2016; 39(2): 258–63.

6   Polonsky WH, Henry RR. Poor medication adherence in type 2 diabetes: recognizing the scope of the problem and its key contributors. *Patient Prefer Adherence*. 2016; 10: 1299–307.

7   Salas M, Hughes D, Zuluaga A, Vardeva K, Lebmeier M. Costs of medication nonadherence in patients with diabetes mellitus: a systematic review and critical analysis of the literature. *Value Health*. 2009; 12(6): 915–22.

8   Capoccia K, Odegard PS, Letassy N. Medication adherence with diabetes medication: a systematic review of the literature. *Diabetes Educ*. 2016; 42(1): 34–71.

9   Gonzalez JS, Peyrot M, McCarl LA, Collins EM, Serpa L, Mimiaga MJ, et al. Depression and diabetes treatment nonadherence: a meta-analysis. *Diabetes Care*. 2008; 31(12): 2398–403.

10 Grenard JL, Munjas BA, Adams JL, Suttorp M, Maglione M, McGlynn EA, et al. Depression and medication adherence in the treatment of chronic diseases in the United States: a meta-analysis. *J Gen Intern Med*. 2011; 26(10): 1175–82.

11 Ali S, Stone MA, Peters JL, Davies MJ, Khunti K. The prevalence of co-morbid depression in adults with type 2 diabetes: a

systematic review and meta-analysis. *Diabet Med*. 2006; 23(11): 1165–73.

12 Detweiler-Bedell JB, Friedman MA, Leventhal H, Miller IW, Leventhal EA. Integrating co-morbid depression and chronic physical disease management: identifying and resolving failures in self-regulation. *Clin Psychol Rev*. 2008; 28(8): 1426–46.

13 Knott C, Bell S, Britton A. Alcohol consumption and the risk of type 2 diabetes: a systematic review and dose-response meta-analysis of more than 1.9 million individuals from 38 observational studies. *Diabetes Care*. 2015; 38(9): 1804–12.

14 Fielding BA, Reid G, Grady M, Humphreys SM, Evans K, Frayn KN. Ethanol with a mixed meal increases postprandial triacylglycerol but decreases postprandial non-esterified fatty acid concentrations. *Br J Nutr*. 2000; 83(6): 597–604.

15 Singh VK, Yadav D, Garg PK. Diagnosis and management of chronic pancreatitis: a review. *JAMA*. 2019; 322(24): 2422–34.

16 Freeman R. Not all neuropathy in diabetes is of diabetic etiology: differential diagnosis of diabetic neuropathy. *Curr Diab Rep*. 2009; 9(6): 423–31.

17 Wakabayashi I, Kobaba-Wakabayashi R, Masuda H. Relation of drinking alcohol to atherosclerotic risk in type 2 diabetes. *Diabetes Care*. 2002; 25(7): 1223–8.

18 van de Wiel A. Diabetes mellitus and alcohol. *Diabetes Metab Res Rev*. 2004; 20 (4): 263–7.

19 Strack F, Deutsch R. Reflective and impulsive determinants of social behavior. *Pers Soc Psychol Rev*. 2004; 8(3): 220–47.

20 Leventhal H, Phillips LA, Burns E. The common-sense model of self-regulation of health and illness. *Self-Regul Health Illn Behav*. 2003; 1: 42–65.

21 Harvey JN, Lawson VL. The importance of health belief models in determining self-care behaviour in diabetes. *Diabet Med*. 2009; 26(1): 5–13.

22 Alison Phillips L, Leventhal H, Leventhal EA. Assessing theoretical predictors of long-term medication adherence: patients' treatment-related beliefs, experiential feedback and habit development. *Psychol Health*. 2013; 28(10): 1135–51.

23 Horne R, Weinman J. Patients' beliefs about prescribed medicines and their role in adherence to treatment in chronic physical illness. *J Psychosom Res*. 1999; 47 (6): 555–67.

24 Horne R, Chapman SC, Parham R, Freemantle N, Forbes A, Cooper V. Understanding patients' adherence-related beliefs about medicines prescribed for long-term conditions: a meta-analytic review of the Necessity-Concerns Framework. *PLoS ONE*. 2013; 8(12): e80633.

25 Verplanken B. Beyond frequency: habit as mental construct. *Br J Soc Psychol*. 2006; 45 (Pt 3): 639–56.

26 O'Carroll R, Whittaker J, Hamilton B, Johnston M, Sudlow C, Dennis M. Predictors of adherence to secondary preventive medication in stroke patients. *Ann Behav Med*. 2011; 41(3): 383–90.

27 O'Carroll RE, Chambers JA, Dennis M, Sudlow C, Johnston M. Improving medication adherence in stroke survivors: mediators and moderators of treatment effects. *Health Psychol*. 2014; 33(10): 1241–50.

28 Wood W, Rünger D. Psychology of habit. *Annu Rev Psychol*. 2016; 67: 289–314.

29 Gardner B. A review and analysis of the use of 'habit' in understanding, predicting and influencing health-related behaviour. *Health Psychol Rev*. 2015; 9(3): 277–95.

30 Phillips LA, Cohen J, Burns E, Abrams J, Renninger S. Self-management of chronic illness: the role of 'habit' versus reflective factors in exercise and medication adherence. *J Behav Med*. 2016; 39(6): 1076–91.

31 Burns RJ, Deschênes SS, Knäuper B, Schmitz N. Habit strength as a moderator of the association between symptoms of poor mental health and unintentional non-adherence to oral hypoglycemic medication in adults with type 2 diabetes. *J Health Psychol*. 2019; 24(3): 321–6.

32 Morisky DE, Ang A, Krousel-Wood M, Ward HJ. Predictive validity of a medication adherence measure in an outpatient setting. *J Clin Hypertens (Greenwich)*. 2008; 10(5): 348–54.

33 Kristensen LJ, Thastum M, Mose AH, Birkebaek NH. Psychometric evaluation of the adherence in diabetes questionnaire. *Diabetes Care*. 2012; 35(11): 2161–6.

34 Toobert DJ, Hampson SE, Glasgow RE. The summary of diabetes self-care activities measure: results from 7 studies and a revised scale. *Diabetes Care*. 2000; 23(7): 943–50.

35 Nunes V, Neilson J, O'Flynn N, Calvert N, Kuntze S, Smithson H, et al. *Clinical Guidelines and Evidence Review for Medicines Adherence: Involving Patients in Decisions about Prescribed Medicines and Supporting Adherence*. National Collaborating Centre for Primary Care and Royal College of General Practitioners, 2009.

36 Binns-Calvey AE, Sharma G, Ashley N, Kelly B, Weaver FM, Weiner SJ. Listening to the patient: a typology of contextual red flags in disease management encounters. *J Patient Cent Res Rev*. 2020; 7 (1): 39–46.

37 Garrett CJ, Choudhary P, Amiel SA, Fonagy P, Ismail K. Recurrent diabetic ketoacidosis and a brief history of brittle diabetes research: contemporary and past evidence in diabetic ketoacidosis research including mortality, mental health and prevention. *Diabet Med*. 2019; 36(11): 1329–35.

38 Zambanini A, Feher MD. Needle phobia in type 1 diabetes mellitus. *Diabet Med*. 1997; 14(4): 321–3.

39 Anderbro T, Amsberg S, Adamson U, Bolinder J, Lins PE, Wredling R, et al. Fear of hypoglycaemia in adults with Type 1 diabetes. *Diabet Med*. 2010; 27(10): 1151–8.

40 Garrett C, Doherty A. Diabetes and mental health. *Clin Med (Lond)*. 2014; 14(6): 669–72.

41 Polonsky W. *Diabetes Burnout: What to Do When You Can't Take It Anymore*. American Diabetes Association, 1999.

42 Todd PJ, Edwards F, Spratling L, Patel NH, Amiel SA, Sturt J, et al. Evaluating the relationships of hypoglycaemia and HbA1c with screening-detected diabetes distress in type 1 diabetes. *Endocrinol Diabetes Metab*. 2018; 1(1): e00003.

43 Horne R, Cooper V, Wileman V, Chan A. Supporting adherence to medicines for long-term conditions. *Eur Psychol*. 2019; 24 (1): 82–96.

44 Horne R, Weinman J, Barber N, Elliott R, Morgan M, Cribb A. *Concordance, Adherence and Compliance in Medicine Taking: Report for the National Co-ordinating Centre for NHS Service Delivery and Organisation*. NHS Service Delivery and Organisation R & D, 2005.

45 Horne R, Weinmann J. The theoretical basis of concordance and issues for research. In: *Concordance: A Partnership in Medicine-Taking* (ed. C Bond). Pharmaceutical Press, 2004, pp. 119–46.

46 Miller WR, Rollnick S. *Motivational Interviewing: Helping People Change*. Guilford Press, 2012.

47 Beck AT, Dozois DJ. Cognitive therapy: current status and future directions. *Annu Rev Med*. 2011; 62: 397–409.

48 DiClemente CC, Velasquez MM. Motivational interviewing and the stages of change. In: *Motivational Interviewing: Preparing People for Change*, 2nd ed. (eds. WR Miller, S Rollnick). Guilford Press, 2002, pp. 201–16.

49 Rollnick S, Allison J. Motivational interviewing. In: *The Essential Handbook of Treatment and Prevention of Alcohol Problems* (eds. N Heather, T Stockwell). John Wiley & Sons, 2004, pp. 105–16.

50 Prochaska JO, DiClemente CC. Toward a comprehensive model of change. In: *Treating Addictive Behaviors* (eds. WR Miller, N Heather). Springer, 1986, pp. 3–27.

51 Schaefer MR, Kavookjian J. The impact of motivational interviewing on adherence and symptom severity in adolescents and young adults with chronic illness: a systematic review. *Patient Educ Couns*. 2017; 100(12): 2190–9.

52 Ismail K, Winkley K, de Zoysa N, Patel A, Heslin M, Graves H, et al. Nurse-led psychological intervention for type 2 diabetes: a cluster randomised controlled trial (Diabetes-6 study) in primary care. *Br J Gen Pract*. 2018; 68(673): e531–40.

53 Ismail K, Maissi E, Thomas S, Chalder T, Schmidt U, Bartlett J, et al. A randomised controlled trial of cognitive behaviour therapy and motivational interviewing for people with type 1 diabetes mellitus with persistent sub-optimal glycaemic control: a Diabetes and Psychological Therapies (ADaPT) study. *Health Technol Assess*. 2010; 14(22): 1–101, iii–iv.

54 Ismail K, Winkley K, Rabe-Hesketh S. Systematic review and meta-analysis of randomised controlled trials of psychological interventions to improve glycaemic control in patients with type 2 diabetes. *Lancet*. 2004; 363(9421): 1589–97.

55 Winkley K, Ismail K, Landau S, Eisler I. Psychological interventions to improve glycaemic control in patients with type 1 diabetes: systematic review and meta-analysis of randomised controlled trials. *BMJ*. 2006; 333(7558): 65.

56 Winkley K, Upsher R, Stahl D, Pollard D, Brennan A, Heller S, et al. Systematic review and meta-analysis of randomized controlled trials of psychological interventions to improve glycaemic control in children and adults with type 1 diabetes. *Diabet Med*. 2020; 37(5): 735–46.

57 Winkley K, Upsher R, Stahl D, Pollard D, Kasera A, Brennan A, et al. Psychological interventions to improve self-management of type 1 and type 2 diabetes: a systematic review. *Health Technol Assess*. 2020; 24(28): 1–232.

58 Winkley K, Upsher R, Stahl D, Pollard D, Brennan A, Heller SR, et al. Psychological interventions to improve glycemic control in adults with type 2 diabetes: a systematic review and meta-analysis. *BMJ Open Diabetes Res Care*. 2020; 8(1): e001150.

Cognitive Impairment and Endocrine Conditions

Anne M. Doherty and Seán F. Dinneen

Introduction

Cognitive impairment or dementia is increasing in prevalence worldwide and may be an unrecognised and early complication of a number of endocrine conditions, including diabetes mellitus and thyroid disease. In addition, these conditions may be predisposing factors towards developing dementia. Identifying cognitive impairments among people with endocrine disorders is important, as is identifying endocrine conditions in people living with dementia. There are particular challenges that present in certain clinical groups, including patients with depressive pseudodementia, behavioural and psychological symptoms of dementia (BPSD), frailty and mild cognitive impairment (MCI). In this chapter, we will discuss these issues with reference to diabetes in particular, being the endocrine disorder with the strongest association with cognitive impairment.

Epidemiology and Aetiology of Cognitive Impairment

Dementia is a neurodegenerative disorder characterised by decline across several domains of cognition, including memory, speech and behaviour, which impacts on functioning. It affects over 46 million people internationally, and this number is projected to rise to over 130 million by 2050: this increase is associated with increased longevity and a worldwide trend towards population ageing (1). Dementia is a heterogeneous condition encompassing a range of conditions and with a range of aetiologies (2).

Alzheimer's disease and vascular dementia are the most common forms of dementia. In addition, there are a range of less common dementias including fronto-temporal dementia (Pick's disease), dementia with Lewy bodies and the dementias secondary to other diseases including AIDS dementia, Parkinson's dementia and alcohol-related brain damage. The key clinical characteristics of each of the principal forms of dementia are outlined in Table 8.1.

Diabetes increases the risk of developing dementia by up to 60%, and diabetes may present for the first time in a person with cognitive impairment or dementia (3). Type 2 diabetes in common in older adults, affecting nearly a fifth of the over 65s, and rising to up to 27% in residential care settings (3, 4). Diabetes is present at similar rates in mental health settings for older adults, with a prevalence of 20% and an estimated 13% of patients having undiagnosed diabetes (5). In a systematic review of the effects of prior hypoglycaemia on cognition in type 1 diabetes, Chandran et al. confirmed that severe hypoglycaemia is associated with cognitive dysfunction, especially when it occurs in childhood or among individuals over 55 years of age. Impaired awareness of hypoglycaemia was associated with poorer memory. Non-severe hypoglycaemia was not associated with cognitive dysfunction (6).

Table 8.1 Characteristics of the dementias.

	Alzheimer's disease	Vascular dementia	Dementia with Lewy bodies	Fronto-temporal dementia
Proportion of dementias	50–80%	20–30%	10–20%	10–15%
Onset	Gradual	Abrupt or gradual	Insidious	Insidious
Course	Progressive, gradual	Progressive, stepwise	Progressive, fluctuating	Rapid
Physical symptoms	Apraxia Aphasia	Focal neurological signs Vascular risk factors	Parkinsonism Falls	
Cognitive symptoms	Memory loss Language deficits Visuospatial deficits	Range of cognitive deficits	Fluctuating cognition	Dysexecutive symptoms
Non-cognitive symptoms	Affective disturbances late in course	Affective lability common	Visual hallucinations	Disinhibition Apathy
Imaging	Generalised atrophy	Strokes Lacunar infarcts Microvascular changes	Generalised atrophy	Frontal and temporal atrophy
Pathology	Generalised atrophy Amyloid plaques Neurofibrillary tangles	Strokes Lacunar infarcts	Generalised atrophy Lewy bodies in the cortex and midbrain	Frontal and temporal atrophy Pick cells in the cortex

Diabetes and Cognition

Cognitive impairment is associated with many challenges to diabetes self-management, including difficulties with medication adherence, difficulties attending clinic appointments, poor insulin administration technique and a reduced ability to recognise or self-manage episodes of hypoglycaemia or hyperglycaemia (7). Individuals with cognitive impairment and diabetes who are treated with insulin are significantly more likely to struggle with the correct management of hypoglycaemia or hyperglycaemia and to have difficulty in utilising 'sick-day rules' (i.e. administering the correct insulin doses for intercurrent illness) (7).

Hypoglycaemia is a serious problem in older adults as it can contribute to an increased risk of falls and death. Over 15,000 hospital admissions in England and Wales annually are due to hypoglycaemia in people aged 60 years and over. The majority of cases have type 2

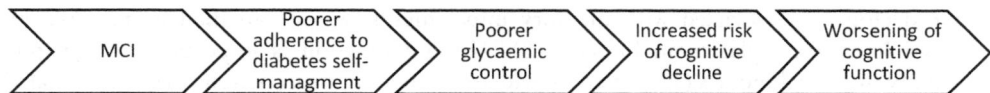

Figure 8.1 Mild cognitive impairment (MCI), dementia and diabetes.

diabetes, and the hypoglycaemia is attributed in these cases to polypharmacy of anti-diabetic agents, altered eating habits and poor nutrition (8–10). Nutritional compromise is a significant difficulty in severe mental illness, with audit data showing that 15% of female inpatients in mental health settings are underweight (body mass index < 18 kg/m^2), which may have an impact on insulin requirements (11).

Mild Cognitive Impairment

MCI is regarded as a prodrome of dementia: at this stage, there is evidence of some mild clinical symptoms that may include both memory and neuropsychiatric symptoms (12). It is estimated to affect as many as 20% of adults aged over 65 years and is associated with a high rate of progression to dementia – up to 10% per year. This is a diagnosable stage of the condition (similar to prediabetes) and is amenable to early intervention. In considering a diagnosis of MCI, a clinician will assess the following changes: subjective cognitive decline or impairment and objective evidence of impairment across one or more cognitive domains, including memory, executive function, attention, language and visuospatial skills, in the presence of intact functioning and the absence of dementia. There are two MCI subtypes: amnestic MCI (where impairment of memory predominates) and non-amnestic MCI (char-acterised by impairments in cognitive domains other than memory). These subtypes reflect the underlying pathology and may predict clinical outcomes. Amnestic MCI is associated with neurodegenerative pathology and is likely to progress to Alzheimer's disease. Non-amnestic MCI may progress to fronto-temporal dementia (especially where just one frontal domain is impaired) or dementia with Lewy bodies (where there are multiple domains affected). It is thought that either subtype may increase the risk of a future onset of vascular dementia (13).

MCI represents an opportunity to implement pharmacological and non-pharmacological strategies to address cognitive functioning and optimise health. There is evidence that, in addition to controlling cardiovascular risk factors, aerobic exercise in particular may have a role in managing this, and other factors, including mental activity and social engagement, may play a role in delaying progression to dementia (14, 15). The American Academy of Neurology does not recommend the used of acetylcholinesterase inhibitors in the management of MCI as the empirical evidence of slowing progression to dementia is weak, although they note that clinicians may choose to offer this as an off-licence treatment (16).

Diabetes is a risk factor for MCI, and the presence of MCI may challenge the optimal treatment of diabetes, which may result in poorer vascular outcomes, including cognition (Figure 8.1). Therefore, it may be helpful for diabetes clinicians to consider cognitive screening in older patients with diabetes and also to consider optimising brain health in this population.

Cognition and Other Endocrine Disorders

Thyroid disorders can be associated with cognitive impairment that may be at least partly reversible with correction of the thyroid abnormality (17). Hypothyroidism induced by thyroidectomy is associated with memory impairments, which can then be reversed by thyroid hormone replacement in rats (18). Thyroid function is important for synaptic plasticity in animal models (19). There is evidence that adult neurogenesis may be regulated via thyroid receptors (TR-alpha), especially in the hippocampus, and that thyroid hormone levels may be involved in this process (20). Hippocampal neurogenesis is thought to play a role in memory, and this may be the mechanism by which thyroid hormone levels influence cognition (21). It has been suggested that thyroid hormone may control the expression of *ChAT*, the gene responsible for acetylcholine synthesis (22). Hashimoto's encephalopathy is a controversial and poorly understood condition characterised by cognitive dysfunction (in addition to seizures, movement disorders and neuropsychiatric symptoms) associated with thyroid peroxidase antibodies in patients who are euthyroid (23). There is weak evidence that parathyroid dysfunction may also be related to cognitive impairment, but it is difficult to draw clear conclusions on this as the evidence is limited by the poor quality of the studies in this area (24). Further detail on the relationship between thyroid and parathyroid dysfunction and mental health symptoms is provided in Chapter 6.

Investigating Cognitive Impairment

The Assessment

Conducting an assessment of dementia involves taking a full history, taking a collateral history, performing an assessment of cognitive status and conducting any appropriate investigations. It is especially important to identify and treat any reversible causes of cognitive impairment. Ideally, this will occur in a specialist memory clinic, but many patients with diabetes and other endocrine disorders present in other non-specialist settings, such as acute medical inpatient units, acute psychiatry settings and psychiatry continuing care settings, where there may be limited availability of specialist input.

History and Examination

Evaluation of cognitive impairment includes a thorough history of the evolution of memory difficulties from the patient – in addition to cognitive symptoms, any behavioural or psychological symptoms should be elicited if possible (25). It is important to obtain a history from a family member or carer and from the patient's primary care doctor (if in secondary care), as the patient may not recall or have full insight into the extent of their difficulties. The person's premorbid functioning is important to interpreting cognitive testing. For example, the 74-year-old retired professor who reads five books a week with a Mini-Mental State Examination (MMSE) of 24 is likely to have had a significantly greater deviation from baseline and more advanced findings on neuroimaging than an age-equivalent counterpart who left school at 12 with a likely borderline learning disability, for whom a score of 24 of the MMSE may not be far from baseline. This concept of *cognitive reserve* accounts for differences in how individuals manifest the symptoms of dementia, especially in Alzheimer's disease, and it is moderated in the main by levels of educational attainment and lifestyle factors. In individuals with a higher cognitive reserve, the brain is able to cope with damage by utilising compensatory mechanisms and a range of pre-existing cognitive processing techniques (26).

It is important to review the medications for any associated anticholinergic burden or other medications that might contribute to cognitive impairment. Unfortunately, these medications are frequently prescribed in older patients (27). A wide range of medications, including antihistamines (H1 blockers), tricyclic antidepressants (more likely now to be prescribed for pain, including pain due to diabetic neuropathy, than for depression), benzodiazepines, anti-muscarinics and opiates, were found to be associated with acute or chronic cognitive impairment in Tannenbaum et al.'s systematic review (28).

It is similarly important to assess mood, as depression is a common cause of reversible cognitive impairment.

Instruments

There are a number of tests recommended by National Institute of Health and Care Excellence (NICE) guidelines for the non-specialist setting, which include the 10-point cognitive screener (10-CS), the 6-item cognitive impairment test (6CIT), the 6-item screener, the Memory Impairment Screen (MIS), the Mini-Cog and the Test Your Memory (TYM) (25). A normal score does not rule out dementia.

Folstein's MMSE and the Montreal Cognitive Assessment (MoCA) are probably the two most commonly used measures in non-specialist settings. Both are 1-page, 10-minute, 30-point cognitive tests. The MMSE has a cut-off of 24 and has a sensitivity of 87%, but it has some limitations. Its sensitivity drops in more highly educated persons to 69%, probably due to the moderating effect of cognitive reserve (26, 29). It does not provide any assessment of executive function and has poor sensitivity in MCI, dementia with Lewy bodies and fronto-temporal dementia (FTD) (30). The cut-off for the MoCA is 26: it is highly sensitive for MCI (94% sensitivity), as well as dementia with Lewy bodies and fronto-temporal dementia (31).

Investigations

Blood investigations should include tests for reversible causes of cognitive decline, including thyroid function tests, folate, vitamin B_{12} and vitamin D, in addition to a full blood count, urea, electrolytes, renal function and liver function. Urine dipstick and culture are more important in excluding a delirium rather than in diagnosing a dementia, but they are essential components of the workup.

Neuroimaging is essential to the workup. Structural magnetic resonance imaging (MRI) will identify medial temporal and hippocampal atrophy, which are suggestive of Alzheimer's disease, and these changes may be present before the full clinical syndrome is evident. The presence of infarcts and white matter hyperintensities in deep white matter on MRI may suggest vascular dementia (32). Neuroimaging also allows for the detection of conditions such as normal-pressure hydrocephalus, where the cognitive impairment is reversible with neurosurgical intervention. Other neuroimaging techniques such as diffusion MRI, single-photon emission computerized tomography (SPECT) and positron emission tomography (PET) scans are less readily available outside the specialist setting.

Rule Out Delirium

Delirium is an acute state of cognitive impairment and global cerebral dysfunction due to a range of insults, including but not limited to intercurrent infection, metabolic dysfunction, etc., and it is characterised by fluctuations in consciousness with deficits in attention,

Table 8.2 Differentiating between depressive pseudodementia and dementia.

	Cognitive impairment associated with depression	Dementia
Onset	Sudden	Gradual
Progression	Rapid	Slow
Insight	Present	Absent
Mood	Depressed	May be incongruous
Vegetative symptoms (e.g. weight loss, anorexia, insomnia)	Common	Rare
Psychiatric history	Frequently present	Less frequently present
On cognitive testing	'I don't know' answers	Makes effort to answer
Suicide risk	Medium to high	Low
Nocturnal exacerbation of symptoms	No	Frequently present

Adapted from Perini et al. (37).

arousal and cognition. It is common in the acute hospital setting, where rates among the elderly can be as high as 89% (33). It may also occur in younger age groups, especially where there is severe illness (e.g. in intensive care settings) (34).

Delirium may be superimposed on dementia, but it is not ideal to assess for dementia in the immediate aftermath of an episode of delirium, as it may take a number of weeks for cognitive function to return to baseline. Delirium increases the risk of developing dementia in the future (35).

Additional Considerations in Dementia

Depressive Pseudodementia

In some cases, cognitive decline may be secondary to a severe depressive illness. In a study that compared patients with late-onset depression and those with Alzheimer's disease, da Silva Novaretti et al. found similar deficits across several cognitive domains, especially in language tasks (36). Perini et al. suggest some key factors that may aid in differentiating between the two conditions, including speed of onset and progression, insight into deficits and mood (Table 8.2) (37). It may be difficult to rule out dementia until the depressive episode is remitted, although cognitive symptoms may persist in a minority of cases (38). The relationship between depression and dementia is complicated as a history of depression increases the risk of future dementia (39, 40), although reversible and irreversible deficits may coexist (41). Depressive pseudodementia is treatable with antidepressants, non-pharmacological treatments and, in some instances, electroconvulsive therapy.

Frailty

Frailty is an increasingly recognised and common syndrome in older adults and is associated with an increased risk of poorer outcomes, including falls and fractures, disability, hospitalisation and mortality (42). Fried et al.'s original phenotypic description defined it as follows: weight loss > 4.5 kg in the past year; reductions in energy, walking speed and physical activity; and weakness as defined by grip strength (43). A subsequent deficit model developed by Rockwood described it as an accumulation of deficits or comorbidities that together lower the person's reserve for further insult and confer greater risk (44). An important concept in considering frailty is that of a time window during which progression to long-term disability can be averted if the underlying condition(s) causing the frailty can be treated. Diabetes is known to be associated with 'accelerated ageing' and is one such treatable condition. There are a number of well-validated measures for assessing frailty. There is evidence that the presence of diabetes increases the risk of frailty, and certainly if Rockwood's accumulation of deficits model is used, it is a key comorbidity. In acknowledgement of the impact of diabetes on frail older adults, the Joint British Diabetes Societies (JBDS) published guidelines for the care of older adults with diabetes and frailty in inpatient settings (45).

Behavioural and Psychological Symptoms of Dementia/Non-cognitive Symptoms

BPSD or non-cognitive symptoms are common in dementia and include disturbance of mood, behaviour, thought or perception, and they may take the form of depression, anxiety, agitation, paranoia, hallucinations, etc. These may have a more profound effect than cognitive difficulties on the person's functioning and quality of life. They are associated with significant carer distress and are predictors of nursing home admission (46). They may affect as many as 80% of people living with dementia at some point in their illness (47). Multiple studies and systematic reviews have found that there is good evidence for the use of non-pharmacological interventions in BPSD, including behavioural management techniques, sensory stimulation interventions and multicomponent therapies (46). The evidence for pharmacological treatments is variable, and there are concerns regarding the safety of psychotropics in particular in this population: they carry a US Food and Drugs Administration (FDA) 'black box' warning in this population (48). A recent systematic review by Yunusa et al. found that atypical antipsychotics are effective in the management of the symptoms of agitation and psychosis in dementia, and this may represent a 'trade-off' against the existing safety concerns in certain cases (49). In patients with diabetes, the use of atypical antipsychotics may have an impact on glycaemic control, similarly to that in younger populations with psychosis (see Chapter 3); however, the optimal management of BPSD may facilitate diabetes management (due to improved cooperation between medications and glucose testing), representing another 'trade-off' against the effects of the antipsychotics.

Fronto-temporal Dementia

Specific difficulties may arise in fronto-temporal dementia, which is frequently associated with hyperorality. This symptom is characterised by the person feeling a compulsion towards placing items in their mouth. This may manifest as increased consumption of cigarettes (increasing vascular risk factors), potomania (which may in severe cases result in water intoxication and electrolyte disturbances, in some instances resulting in seizures) and an increase in the intake of food, especially sweet items (further challenging diabetes management) (50, 51).

Mental Capacity

Capacity is the inherent ability to make an informed decision. A person may have capacity to make one decision but not another, and assessment of capacity is usually decision-specific. All people are presumed to have capacity unless demonstrated otherwise, and those with capacity all have the right to make unwise decisions. Thus, the onus is on the assessor to demonstrate where the deficit in capacity may lie. Capacity may be impaired by a transient illness – either a mental disorder such as a psychotic episode or a physical disorder that impinges on the mind such as a delirium – and in these cases the person may regain capacity. Capacity may also be impaired by a more chronic condition such as dementia, where it is unlikely that the person will regain capacity.

Mental capacity is not always impaired in dementia, but where this is the case it may be important to take measures to ensure the safety of the individual patient. Capacity is rarely assessed in practice unless there is a specific difficulty posed, such as a person not wishing to proceed with treatment or, more frequently, not understanding the degree of their functional impairments and the need for assistance. With respect to mental capacity, the basic concepts on non-maleficence are paramount: avoiding any unavoidable harm that may come to the person and affording what protections are available under the law. If the individual's lack of capacity is not affecting their well-being in any material way, then formal assessment of capacity is not indicated as intervention is not required.

Assessment

Mental capacity is addressed in the law in different ways depending on the legal jurisdiction, with differing remedies and processes recommended in different countries. It is beyond the scope of this book to discuss such differing laws, but we will discuss the overarching principles in brief.

The first question is whether or not the person has a disorder affecting the mind, which may include mental illnesses, dementias or delirium, to name a few. The second question is whether this disorder impacts on the person's ability to make the decision that is in question.

The four tests of capacity are:

(1) The ability to understand the information – this includes understanding the proposed course of action and alternatives, along with the risks and benefits of the various options.
(2) The ability to retain the information.
(3) The ability to weigh the information in the balance – this is the process of actual decision-making. Here, one might consider what factors are influencing the person's decision.
(4) The ability to communicate the decision.

Every possible effort must be made to aid the person in understanding the issues at hand, such as using pictures, videos and examples, ensuring they have their hearing aids, ensuring that translators or sign language interpreters are provided where required and ensuring that the information is provided in as simple and understandable a manner as possible and free of jargon.

Vignette

John, a 71-year-old retired teacher with a 50-year history of type 1 diabetes, has been admitted with diabetic ketoacidosis (DKA). He was diagnosed with Alzheimer's disease three years previously, and approximately two years ago he was under the care of a psychiatry of later life service for BPSD taking the form of agitation and paranoia towards his wife. These symptoms settled quickly with a low dose of atypical antipsychotic (quetiapine 25 mg) and there has been no further concern regarding his mental state. He was admitted four weeks ago with increased confusion and hyperglycaemia, and he was diagnosed with a lower respiratory tract infection and commenced on intravenous antibiotics. John's wife reported that in recent months she was concerned about his diabetes management – in earlier life he had managed this well, but now he seemed confused about when to administer insulin and how to correct abnormal blood glucose levels, giving the example of him trying to correct a blood glucose of 21 with orange juice. He was not willing to allow her to assist him as he felt that he was the expert. His HbA1c on admission was 102 mmol/mol.

During the admission, in the initial phase of illness John would frequently request insulin when it had already been given, but this was attributed to delirium – acute-on-chronic cognitive impairment due to infection. When he was allowed to self-administer insulin on the ward he developed a recurrence of DKA. Due to his wife's concerns and the observed difficulties in self-management in the hospital setting, a meeting was held about John's care into the future. He was adamant that he would manage at home, and a care package was arranged with 20 hours of carer presence per week.

John was discharged home, but he readmitted within 24 hours with hyperglycaemia and ketonaemia.

His wife, in tears, told you she is not able to manage him at home any longer.

What would you like to do now?

Full workup on initial admission showed some microvascular changes and global cerebral atrophy on brain MRI. All bloods (including thyroid function, vitamin B_{12} and folate) were normal once the inflammatory markers settled following resolution of the lower respiratory tract infection. Cognitive testing showed a deterioration from 23/30 (two years previously) to 21/30 on the MoCA, with deficits in short-term memory and executive function.

John is unwilling to accept the idea of residential care, but you believe he lacks capacity to manage his diabetes safely. You believe he does not fully understand the risks posed by his cognitive impairment to his diabetes management and general health, and when you explain that he is at risk of death if unsupervised, he does not believe your claim that a higher level of care is required. Therefore, you conclude that he is unable to weigh 'in the balance' the factors affecting the decision about his care.

You request a second opinion from your geriatric health colleagues. They agree with you, and together you initiate your country-specific legal mechanism to protect John's rights while ensuring his safety.

Management

Adherence

Managing dementia and diabetes when they coexist can be a considerable challenge. Some patients will have had good premorbid adherence, but memory problems may now pose a significant barrier to adherence in the presence of dementia. Other patients will have had poorer premorbid adherence. Regardless of premorbid adherence, it will be important to find solutions to adherence in later life, especially where there is comorbid cognitive impairment. Reminders of various forms may aid adherence to oral medications and insulin alike – these may take the form of blister packs, alarms and calendars, or perhaps prompting by a family member or carer (52).

Avoiding Hypoglycaemia and Falls

Hypoglycaemia is associated with many adverse outcomes, including further deterioration in cognitive status, cardiovascular and cerebrovascular events, malnutrition, falls and associated increased mortality and death (53). Falls are associated with fractures (reduced bone density associated with diabetes being an additional risk factor), and hip fractures in particular are associated with poorer outcomes in older adults: mortality rates in the year following a hip fracture are high (54) and may result in adverse outcomes in terms of mood and quality of life, with few patients returning to premorbid functioning (55).

Less tight HbA1c targets may be required, although the degree to which they should be relaxed is not universally agreed upon. The American Diabetes Association recommends a target HbA1c of <7.5% (59 mmol/mol) for older adults with intact cognition, the American Association of Clinical Endocrinologists recommends <6.5% (58 mmol/mol) if it can be achieved safely, with less tight targets for patients with concurrent illnesses or at risk of hypoglycaemia, and the American College of Physicians suggests 7–8% (53–64 mmol/mol) for older adults (56). The 2020 Guidelines of the American Diabetes Association recommend a less stringent HbA1c goal (e.g. <64 mmol/mol or 8%) in selected patients such as those with extensive comorbid conditions (57). The International Diabetes Federation has devised a categorical framework recommending targets of 7.0–7.5% (53–59 mmol/mol) in the functionally independent and 7.0–8.0% (53–64 mmol/mol) in the functionally dependent. For vulnerable categories (e.g. dementia and frailty), the International Diabetes Federation recommends as high as 8.5% (70 mmol/mol), and in end-of-life care the aim is simply to avoid symptomatic hyperglycaemia (58).

Clinical Pathways

A UK-based national expert group produced a best clinical practice statement that suggested principles of care for people with diabetes and dementia, emphasised the importance of having well-defined clinical pathways for the integration of care for this population and promoted earlier detection of both diabetes in dementia and dementia in diabetes (8). This is important not just in the community but also in long-term mental health facilities and other residential care settings, where there are higher rates of comorbidities.

Practical Considerations

Many older adults with cognitive impairment may find small, 'fiddly' devices for finger pricking and testing and even insulin pens to be difficult due to the challenges in manual dexterity associated with cognitive decline, apraxia or dyspraxia. Where visual impairment is present (and this is more likely in older adults with diabetes due to the higher risk of diabetic retinopathy and maculopathy in addition to the usual presbyopia of ageing), this may further challenge the use of these devices, which presents particular risks when there is difficulty in seeing the details on insulin pens (52). These difficulties may be addressed to a limited degree by using large-display glucose monitors and insulin pens.

An occupational therapy assessment may be useful in assessing difficulties in manual dexterity. Where there is evidence of difficulties, it may be necessary to consider what provisions need to be made to overcome any difficulties relating to visual impairment or apraxia. Is there someone living with the patient who might be in a position to assist with glucose monitoring and insulin administration? If not, are there family members nearby who can assist reliably? Does home care need to be arranged? We are only beginning to appreciate the challenges associated with managing diabetes in the frail, elderly populations that are becoming an increasingly common part of our healthcare systems throughout the developed world. A combined effort between diabetology and geriatric medicine (similar to that see in orthogeriatrics services) will probably be required in order to address these challenges.

Conclusion

Cognitive impairment or dementia is increasing in prevalence worldwide, and it is important to identify this in those with pre-existing endocrine disorders, especially diabetes. These conditions also increase the risk of developing cognitive impairment. Identifying cognitive impairments among people with endocrine disorders is important, as is identifying endocrine conditions in people living with dementia, as the presence of these may require adjustment of therapeutic targets and of treatment. There are particular challenges in certain clinical groups, including depressive pseudodementia, BPSD, frailty and MCI. Targets for glycaemic control may need to be relaxed in this group of patients, and this is supported by international best practice guidelines.

References

1   Alzheimer's Disease International. *World Alzheimer's Report 2015: The Global Impact of Dementia*. Alzheimer's Disease International, 2015.

2   Gale SA, Acar D, Daffner KR. Dementia. *Am J Med.* 2018; 131(10): 1161–9.

3   Chatterjee S, Peters SA, Woodward M, Mejia Arango S, Batty GD, Beckett N, et al. Type 2 diabetes as a risk factor for dementia in women compared with men: a pooled analysis of 2.3 million people comprising more than 100,000 cases of dementia. *Diabetes Care.* 2016; 39(2): 300–7.

4   Fagot-Campagna A, Bourdel-Marchasson I, Simon D. Burden of diabetes in an aging population: prevalence, incidence, mortality, characteristics and quality of care. *Diabetes Metab.* 2005; 31(Spec. No. 2): 5s35–52.

5   Aspray TJ, Nesbit K, Cassidy TP, Farrow E, Hawthorne G. Diabetes in British nursing and residential homes: a pragmatic screening study. *Diabetes Care.* 2006; 29(3): 707–8.

6   Chandran SR, Jacob P, Choudhary P. A systematic review of the effect of prior hypoglycaemia on cognitive function in type 1 diabetes. *Ther Adv Endocrinol Metab.* 2020; 11: 2042018820906017.

7   Tomlin A, Sinclair A. The influence of cognition on self-management of type 2 diabetes in older people. *Psychol Res Behav Manag.* 2016; 9: 7–20.

8   Sinclair AJ, Hillson R, Bayer AJ. Diabetes and dementia in older people: a Best Clinical Practice Statement by a multidisciplinary National Expert Working Group. *Diabet Med.* 2014; 31(9): 1024–31.

9   Bunn F, Goodman C, Malone JR, Jones PR, Burton C, Rait G, et al. Managing diabetes in people with dementia: protocol for a realist review. *Syst Rev.* 2016; 5: 5.

10   Salutini E, Bianchi C, Santini M, Dardano A, Daniele G, Penno G, et al. Access to emergency room for hypoglycaemia in people with diabetes. *Diabetes Metab Res Rev.* 2015; 31(7): 745–51.

11   JBDS, RCPsych. *The Management of Diabetes in Adults and Children with Psychiatric Disorders in Inpatient Settings.* Joint British Diabetes Societies and Royal College of Psychiatrists, 2017.

12   Dubois B, Feldman HH, Jacova C, Cummings JL, Dekosky ST, Barberger-Gateau P, et al. Revising the definition of Alzheimer's disease: a new lexicon. *Lancet Neurol.* 2010; 9(11): 1118–27.

13   Roberts R, Knopman DS. Classification and epidemiology of MCI. *Clin Geriatr Med.* 2013; 29(4): 753–72.

14   Devenney KE, Guinan EM, Kelly AM, Mota BC, Walsh C, Olde Rikkert M, et al. Acute high-intensity aerobic exercise affects brain-derived neurotrophic factor in mild cognitive impairment: a randomised controlled study. *BMJ Open Sport Exerc Med.* 2019; 5(1): e000499.

15   Langa KM, Levine DA. The diagnosis and management of mild cognitive impairment: a clinical review. *JAMA.* 2014; 312(23): 2551–61.

16   Petersen RC, Lopez O, Armstrong MJ, Getchius TSD, Ganguli M, Gloss D, et al. Practice guideline update summary: mild cognitive impairment: report of the Guideline Development, Dissemination, and Implementation Subcommittee of the American Academy of Neurology. *Neurology.* 2018; 90(3): 126–35.

17   Mistry N, Wass J, Turner MR. When to consider thyroid dysfunction in the neurology clinic. *Pract Neurol.* 2009; 9(3): 145–56.

18   Alzoubi KH, Gerges NZ, Aleisa AM, Alkadhi KA. Levothyroxin restores hypothyroidism-induced impairment of hippocampus-dependent learning and memory: behavioral, electrophysiological, and molecular studies. *Hippocampus.* 2009; 19(1): 66–78.

19   Vara H, Martinez B, Santos A, Colino A. Thyroid hormone regulates neurotransmitter release in neonatal rat hippocampus. *Neuroscience.* 2002; 110(1): 19–28.

20   Kapoor R, van Hogerlinden M, Wallis K, Ghosh H, Nordstrom K, Vennstrom B, et al. Unliganded thyroid hormone receptor alpha1 impairs adult hippocampal neurogenesis. *FASEB J.* 2010; 24(12): 4793–805.

21   Shors TJ, Townsend DA, Zhao M, Kozorovitskiy Y, Gould E. Neurogenesis may relate to some but not all types of hippocampal-dependent learning. *Hippocampus.* 2002; 12(5): 578–84.

22   Leach PT, Gould TJ. Thyroid hormone signaling: contribution to neural function, cognition, and relationship to nicotine. *Neurosci Biobehav Rev.* 2015; 57: 252–63.

23   Montagna G, Imperiali M, Agazzi P, D'Aurizio F, Tozzoli R, Feldt-Rasmussen U, et al. Hashimoto's encephalopathy: a rare proteiform disorder. *Autoimmun Rev.* 2016; 15(5): 466–76.

24   Lourida I, Thompson-Coon J, Dickens CM, Soni M, Kuźma E, Kos K, et al. Parathyroid hormone, cognitive function and dementia: a systematic review. *PLoS ONE.* 2015; 10 (5): e0127574.

25   NICE. *Dementia: Assessment, Management and Support for People Living with Dementia and Their Carers (NICE Guideline NG97).* National Institute for Health and Care Excellence, 2018.

26   Stern Y. Cognitive reserve in ageing and Alzheimer's disease. *Lancet Neurol.* 2012; 11(11): 1006–12.

27   Green AR, Reifler LM, Boyd CM, Weffald LA, Bayliss EA. Medication profiles of patients with cognitive impairment and high anticholinergic burden. *Drugs Aging.* 2018; 35(3): 223–32.

28 Tannenbaum C, Paquette A, Hilmer S, Holroyd-Leduc J, Carnahan R. A systematic review of amnestic and non-amnestic mild cognitive impairment induced by anticholinergic, antihistamine, GABAergic and opioid drugs. *Drugs Aging.* 2012; 29(8): 639–58.

29 Kang JM, Cho YS, Park S, Lee BH, Sohn BK, Choi CH, et al. Montreal Cognitive Assessment reflects cognitive reserve. *BMC Geriatr.* 2018; 18(1): 261.

30 Velayudhan L, Ryu SH, Raczek M, Philpot M, Lindesay J, Critchfield M, et al. Review of brief cognitive tests for patients with suspected dementia. *Int Psychogeriatr.* 2014; 26(8): 1247–62.

31 Luis CA, Keegan AP, Mullan M. Cross validation of the Montreal Cognitive Assessment in community dwelling older adults residing in the southeastern US. *Int J Geriatr Psychiatry.* 2009; 24(2): 197–201.

32 Ruan Q, D'Onofrio G, Sancarlo D, Bao Z, Greco A, Yu Z. Potential neuroimaging biomarkers of pathologic brain changes in mild cognitive impairment and Alzheimer's disease: a systematic review. *BMC Geriatr.* 2016; 16: 104.

33 Fick DM, Agostini JV, Inouye SK. Delirium superimposed on dementia: a systematic review. *J Am Geriatr Soc.* 2002; 50(10): 1723–32.

34 Krewulak KD, Stelfox HT, Ely EW, Fiest KM. Risk factors and outcomes among delirium subtypes in adult ICUs: a systematic review. *J Crit Care.* 2020; 56: 257–64.

35 Witlox J, Eurelings LS, de Jonghe JF, Kalisvaart KJ, Eikelenboom P, van Gool WA. Delirium in elderly patients and the risk of postdischarge mortality, institutionalization, and dementia: a meta-analysis. *JAMA.* 2010; 304(4): 443–51.

36 da Silva Novaretti TM, D'Avila Freitas MI, Mansur LL, Nitrini R, Radanovic M. Comparison of language impairment in late-onset depression and Alzheimer's disease. *Acta Neuropsychiatr.* 2011; 23(2): 62–8.

37 Perini G, Cotta Ramusino M, Sinforiani E, Bernini S, Petrachi R, Costa A. Cognitive impairment in depression: recent advances and novel treatments. *Neuropsychiatr Dis Treat.* 2019; 15: 1249–58.

38 Conradi HJ, Ormel J, de Jonge P. Presence of individual (residual) symptoms during depressive episodes and periods of remission: a 3-year prospective study. *Psychol Med.* 2011; 41(6): 1165–74.

39 Diniz BS, Butters MA, Albert SM, Dew MA, Reynolds CF, 3rd. Late-life depression and risk of vascular dementia and Alzheimer's disease: systematic review and meta-analysis of community-based cohort studies. *Br J Psychiatry.* 2013; 202(5): 329–35.

40 Saez-Fonseca JA, Lee L, Walker Z. Long-term outcome of depressive pseudodementia in the elderly. *J Affect Disord.* 2007; 101(1–3): 123–9.

41 McAllister TW, Price TR. Severe depressive pseudodementia with and without dementia. *Am J Psychiatry.* 1982; 139(5): 626–9.

42 Theou O, Sluggett JK, Bell JS, Lalic S, Cooper T, Robson L, et al. Frailty, hospitalization, and mortality in residential aged care. *J Gerontol A Biol Sci Med Sci.* 2018; 73(8): 1090–6.

43 Fried LP, Tangen CM, Walston J, Newman AB, Hirsch C, Gottdiener J, et al. Frailty in older adults: evidence for a phenotype. *J Gerontol A Biol Sci Med Sci.* 2001; 56(3): M146–56.

44 Rockwood K. Conceptual models of frailty: accumulation of deficits. *Can J Cardiol.* 2016; 32(9): 1046–50.

45 JBDS. *Inpatient Care of the Frail Older Adult with Diabetes.* Joint British Diabetes Societies, 2019.

46 Abraha I, Rimland JM, Trotta FM, Dell'Aquila G, Cruz-Jentoft A, Petrovic M, et al. Systematic review of systematic reviews of non-pharmacological interventions to treat behavioural disturbances in older patients with dementia. The SENATOR-OnTop series. *BMJ Open.* 2017; 7(3): e012759.

47 Ryu SH, Katona C, Rive B, Livingston G. Persistence of and changes in neuropsychiatric symptoms in Alzheimer

disease over 6 months: the LASER-AD study. *Am J Geriatr Psychiatry.* 2005; 13 (11): 976–83.

48   Meeks TW, Jeste DV. Beyond the black box: what is the role for antipsychotics in dementia? *Curr Psychiatr.* 2008; 7(6): 50–65.

49   Yunusa I, Alsumali A, Garba AE, Regestein QR, Eguale T. Assessment of reported comparative effectiveness and safety of atypical antipsychotics in the treatment of behavioral and psychological symptoms of dementia: a network meta-analysis. *JAMA Netw Open.* 2019; 2(3): e190828.

50   Hamdy RC, Kinser A, Dickerson K, Kendall-Wilson T, Depelteau A, Whalen K. Fronto-temporal dementia, diabetes mellitus and excessive eating. *Gerontol Geriatr Med.* 2018; 4: 2333721418777057.

51   Rascovsky K, Hodges JR, Knopman D, Mendez MF, Kramer JH, Neuhaus J, et al. Sensitivity of revised diagnostic criteria for the behavioural variant of frontotemporal dementia. *Brain.* 2011; 134(Pt 9): 2456–77.

52   Hillson R. *Diabetes Care: A Practical Manual.* Oxford University Press, 2008.

53   Bruce DG, Davis WA, Casey GP, Clarnette RM, Brown SG, Jacobs IG, et al. Severe hypoglycaemia and cognitive impairment in older patients with diabetes: the Fremantle Diabetes Study. *Diabetologia.* 2009; 52(9): 1808–15.

54   Vestergaard P, Rejnmark L, Mosekilde L. Increased mortality in patients with a hip fracture – effect of pre-morbid conditions and post-fracture complications. *Osteoporos Int.* 2007; 18 (12): 1583–93.

55   Alexiou KI, Roushias A, Varitimidis SE, Malizos KN. Quality of life and psychological consequences in elderly patients after a hip fracture: a review. *Clin Interv Aging.* 2018; 13: 143–50.

56   Longo M, Bellastella G, Maiorino MI, Meier JJ, Esposito K, Giugliano D. Diabetes and aging: from treatment goals to pharmacologic therapy. *Front Endocrinol (Lausanne).* 2019; 10: 45.

57   American Diabetes Association. 6. Glycemic targets: standards of medical care in diabetes – 2020. *Diabetes Care.* 2020; 43 (Suppl. 1): S66–76.

58   Sinclair A, Dunning T, Colagiuri S. *IDF Global Guidelines for Managing Older People with Type 2 Diabetes.* International Diabetes Federation, 2019.

Chapter 9

Suicidal Ideation and Self-Harm

Anne M. Doherty and Seán F. Dinneen

Introduction

Suicide is a leading cause of death in many Western countries. Suicidal ideation and behaviours can be symptoms of depression, but they are also seen in people with other mental health problems, such as bipolar affective disorder, psychosis, substance abuse disorders and adjustment disorders. They are also seen in people who present with psychological distress rather than any diagnosable mental disorder. The consequences of suicidal acts may be especially serious in people with diabetes given the accessibility of lethal means, on the one hand, but also the heightened risk of developing complications in cases of severe self-neglect due to a more passive death wish. In Chapter 2, we discussed the relationship between depression and endocrine disorders. Although depression is associated with suicidal ideations and behaviours, it will be these symptoms rather than a diagnosis of mood disorder that will be the focus of this chapter.

Epidemiology

Suicidality is not a diagnosis, but suicidal ideation and behaviours may be features of a number of psychiatric disorders, and they are important symptoms (indeed, diagnostic criteria) in depression (1). Much of the literature in suicide is not specifically in the area of depression. A seminal paper by Robins et al. published in 1959 described one of the first psychological autopsy studies, which examined the cases of 139 people who died by suicide (a psychological autopsy study attempts to provide a posthumous diagnosis for people who have died by suicide by carrying out a rigorous investigation, reviewing as many sources as possible, including case notes, and interviewing family, professionals and others). The psychological autopsy did not diagnose any of the individuals with a depressive episode, instead identifying a majority with 'manic depressive disorder' or 'chronic alcoholism' (2). A Danish population study of people who died by suicide reported that depressive episode along with borderline personality disorder (BPD) were the psychiatric diagnoses most commonly associated with suicide, although other diagnoses were more common in certain subgroups (3). Data from the UK Confidential Inquiry into homicides and suicides in people with a history of attendance at mental health services found that only 17% had a depressive episode diagnosed prior to death (4). In a systematic review of completed suicide in psychiatric inpatients, Bowers et al. identified previous suicidal behaviour, availability of means, absence of support and the presence of family conflict as variables that increase the risk of suicidal behaviour in depressed psychiatric inpatients (5). A more recent psychological autopsy study in India diagnosed a majority or 54% with depressive episode (6).

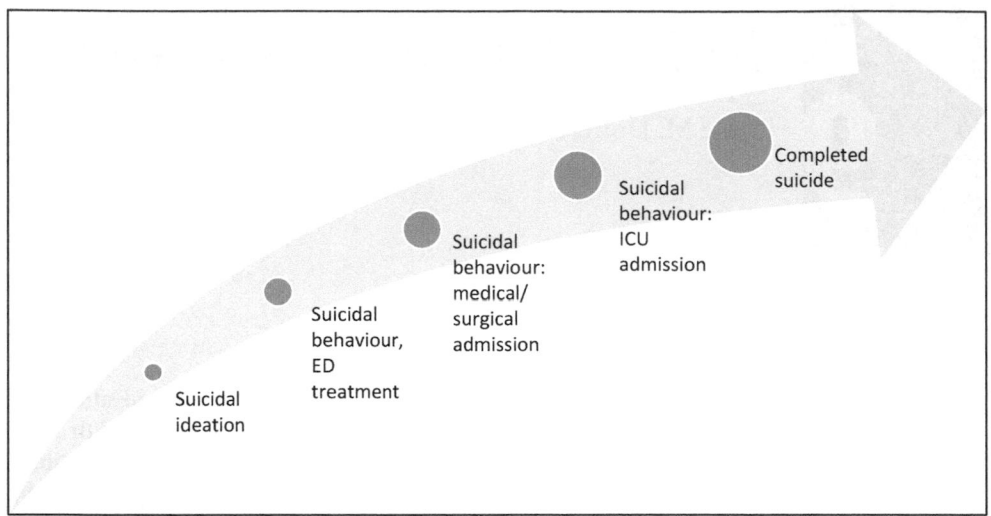

Figure 9.1 Suicidal behaviours as a spectrum along medical severity. ED: emergency department; ICU: intensive care unit. Adapted from Mohan et al. (9)

There is evidence that there may be significant differences between individuals who attempt and those who complete suicide. Significantly higher rates of diagnosed depressive episode have been reported among individuals who completed suicide: 54.9% compared with 27.9% in those who attempted suicide (7). Those individuals who completed suicide were also more likely to be male, to live alone, to describe somatic symptoms prior to the suicidal act and to have recently attended a primary care physician. In a Spanish study that compared individuals who completed suicide with those who attempted suicide, Giner and colleagues noted that male gender, personality disorder, physical health problems and alcohol abuse were significantly more common among those who completed suicide (8). Interesting as these comparisons may be, this style of study comparing living individuals who have attempted suicide (and who are thus available for examination) with those who have died by suicide (regarding whom only retrospective records and collateral reports are available) has inherent biases that are mentioned as limitations in these studies (8).

Suicidality may indeed be seen as a spectrum from passive death wish, through suicidal ideation, self-harm or suicidal behaviours at varying levels of lethality (see Figure 9.1) (9). This model suggests that patients who require hospitalisation, and in particular admission to critical care, may have more features in common with those who die by suicide than patients who express suicidal ideations, although individual patients may be at different points on this spectrum at different times.

Some patients experience difficulty in adjusting to the diagnosis of a new illness, especially if they have already had difficulty in adjustment to the diagnosis of their psychiatric disorder. Distress related to adjustment to a diagnosis of diabetes has been reported in many different settings (10). This may present in different ways in different patients, including non-adherence or the development or escalation of self-injurious behaviours such as repeated self-harm due to psychological distress. Self-harm can be active with obvious suicide attempts (which may involve overdose of insulin or another hypoglycaemic agent) or more occult, manifesting as repeated admissions for diabetic ketoacidosis (DKA) or other medical complications related to diabetes. This may be viewed as ambivalence towards living with diabetes or an indirect suicidal wish. It is possible that adjustment disorders or reactive depression related to the development of diabetes may not always be evident, even to mental health teams, and symptoms may be interpreted as indicators of relapse of their underlying mental illness.

Suicide and Self-Harm in the General Hospital

Not all acts of self-harm are with suicidal intent. It is important not to infer or assume intent, but to ensure that all patients who present with self-harm receive a mental health assessment, in accordance with National Institute for Health and Care Excellence (NICE) guidelines (11). Endocrinologists are most likely to encounter suicidal patients when covering the acute medical services, where any patients presenting with self-harm requiring medical admission will be seen. In the USA, a nationwide emergency department (ED)-based study reported that 0.4% of ED visits over 15 years were due to self-injury, and of those 31% required critical care admission (12). A systematic review of the literature found that there was a strong association between suicidal behaviours and certain diagnoses, including adjustment disorder and depression, in the general hospital setting (13).

The association between the risk of having physical and mental comorbidities is strong and consistent across different settings. It can be difficult, even for specialists, to differentiate Tenth Revision of the International Classification of Disease and Related Health Problems (ICD-10) psychiatric disorders from psychological distress, but there is emerging evidence that both can have a significant effect on physical health outcomes.

Suicide and Self-Harm and Diabetes

Diabetes can present a particular challenge in the management of suicidal ideations and behaviours given that insulin, the essential treatment for type 1 diabetes (and used by many individuals with type 2 diabetes), is potentially lethal in overdose. For example, psychiatrists would generally avoid prescribing medications that can be lethal in overdose, such as tricyclic antidepressants, in patients with a history of suicidal behaviours or current ideations, but in the case of a person with diabetes who requires insulin, this potentially lethal means cannot be easily removed.

Roberts et al. reported that people with type 1 diabetes had a significantly increased rate of suicide, being 11 times greater than that of the general population (14). Subsequent studies have confirmed an elevated rate of suicide among people with diabetes, although not to the same magnitude. Roy et al. found that African-American patients with type 1 diabetes in New Jersey had significantly higher rates (three to four times) of suicide attempts compared with controls without diabetes (13.3% vs 3.5%), and 10% of patients had ongoing suicidal ideation (15). This study reported that, on multivariate analysis, female gender, higher numbers of childhood traumas, depression and alcohol abuse were independently significantly associated with attempted suicide. After controlling for the other factors, each additional type of childhood abuse was associated with an increased risk of attempted suicide of 50%. Those who attempted suicide had higher rates of smoking, alcohol abuse and drug abuse (consistent with the raised risk of suicidal behaviour among people with substance abuse difficulties in the general population).

In a population-based study of completed suicide in northern Finland, Lofman et al. reported that 81% of individuals with type 1 diabetes who had died from suicide by poisoning had previously been hospitalised due to depression, substance abuse or both (16). This study examined all cases of death by suicide (n = 2489) during a 13-year period in northern Finland. The prevalence of hospital-treated diabetes in this suicide population was 3.1%, and 34.6% of them had type 1 diabetes. This study found that almost half of the people with type 1 diabetes who had died from suicide had died by poisoning, a proportion that was over two-times higher than among those without diabetes. Insulin overdose was the cause of death in half of those who died by self-poisoning. Typically, those who died were male and insulin was the only drug used. Insulin was less frequently used as a means of suicide in people with type 2 diabetes who died by suicide, and it was not at all used in people without a diagnosis of diabetes who died by suicide (16).

A study of 100 Italian patients with diabetes demonstrated more severe levels of hopelessness and suicidal ideation than in internal medicine patients, with 23% reporting having had suicidal thoughts (17). This study also reported an association between multiple treatments and hopelessness, although the clinical significance of this relationship is unclear.

A French population-based study examined the incidence of suicidal behaviours (resulting in psychiatric admission) in the years following admission with DKA. It was found that 7.0% of patients with type 1 diabetes and a history of DKA were hospitalised during the nine-year follow-up period compared to 2.5% of individuals with type 1 diabetes and no history of DKA. The rate increased to 16.2% among those patients with type 1 diabetes, previous DKA and a history of mental illness. The rates were highest in the first 12 months following the admission for DKA (18).

In a systematic review, Pompili et al. reported that there may be an especially high risk of suicide among young men with type 1 diabetes, and this was most marked among those between the ages of 15 and 29 years (17). They recommended that physicians should routinely ask their young patients about suicidal thoughts given the relationship of these thoughts with adherence to the medical treatment (17).

Direct Self-Harm

There is a prevalence of intentional overdose of oral hypoglycaemic agents and suicide attempts in people with diabetes of around 15%, and suicidal ideation and passive death wish, perhaps associated with self-neglect, may be even higher. In addition to the risks related to a higher incidence of mental disorders, diabetes mellitus presents specific risks in the ready access to lethal means. Roberts et al. reported that people with type 1 diabetes had a significantly increased rate of suicide: 11 times that of the general population (14). Russell et al. suggested that attempted suicide or suicidal behaviours may explain many of the large numbers of admissions to hospital with unexplained hypoglycaemia, although they note that there are few published data in this area and that the narrow therapeutic index of insulin can make it difficult to attribute intent with certainty in the absence of the patient disclosing their intent (19).

A study of insulin overdoses found that the vast majority (89%) represented acts with some degree of suicidal intent and that the majority presented more than six hours following overdose (20). Insulin pumps in particular present a very simple means of delivering a large and potentially fatal bolus of insulin. In addition, people who use insulin pumps do not receive any long-acting insulins, and being reliant on a constant infusion of short-acting insulins mean that they can die within hours of pump failure (21). Thus, pump removal or sabotage may theoretically be a potential means of suicide, although there are no such reports in the literature.

Every year, a large number of patients with type 1 diabetes present to EDs with hypoglycaemia of unknown aetiology, and it is possible that a significant proportion of them may be intentional overdoses (19). Thus, suicide risk may be underestimated in patients with type 1 diabetes. Boileau et al. were unable to identify any specific feature to predict or recognise secret insulin self-injections (22).

Indirect Self-Harm

In addition to 'direct self-harm' or intentional overdoses of insulin and oral hypoglycaemic agents as suicide attempts in people with diabetes, it is important to consider 'indirect self-harm'. This may include self-neglect (including not taking medications), which may be uncovered when exploring adherence to self-management. It may be associated with low self-esteem, difficulties with motivation and even a passive death wish in depression (23).

DKA is a leading cause of mortality in people with diabetes. If it cannot be explained (i.e. if it is not due to diabetes being undiagnosed, concomitant infection, pump failure, etc.), it may be due to psychosocial factors, and recurrent DKA (rDKA) that is unexplained should trigger a psychosocial assessment (24). Insulin omission is the leading cause of DKA (24). In the past, patients who presented with rDKA were often described as having 'brittle diabetes', and the difficulties of these patients often confounded the best efforts of clinicians and researchers: in some cases, a factitious aetiology was identified as being contributory (25). Bryden et al. reported that having a psychiatric diagnosis predicted DKA, and conversely DKA predicted the development of a mental disorder at 10 years (26). In a study that examined patients with rDKA and compared them to a group of patients with stable diabetes, Pelizza and Pupo found no difference between the two groups in terms of mental illness but significantly higher rates of personality disorders in the 'brittle' group (27). In a review of the literature on 'brittle' diabetes, Garrett et al. noted that while there are clear protocols around the management of recurrent hypoglycaemia, rDKA has fallen out of favour among researchers, and there remains less evidence for the medium/long-term management of the same (28). In adolescents, Goldston et al. found that suicidal thoughts were strongly associated with poor compliance with diabetes self-management (29).

Personality Disorders

BPD, or emotionally unstable personality disorder (EUPD), is a condition characterised by chronic suicidality and often by acts of self-harm, in addition to instability of identity, affect and interpersonal relationships, along with rapidly changing moods, anxiety and dissociative symptoms. It is a truly debilitating condition: people with BPD may be considered to be difficult to engage in treatment and frequently present in crisis (30). As many as 75% of people with BPD engage in self-harm (31), and it has an associated suicide rate of up to 10% (50 times that of the general population) (32).

This diagnosis should only be made by a specialist, and even that with great care, as personality disorders may exist alongside other psychiatric conditions, and people with personality disorders often report a sense of being discriminated against even by healthcare professionals, with some evidence of stigmatising attitudes in this population (33–35). Until the end of the twentieth century, there was a sense of therapeutic nihilism regarding patients with this condition, but the growing evidence base for certain psychological therapies, namely dialectic behaviour therapy and mentalisation-based treatment, has changed the emphasis to one of active treatment (36).

Where BPD is suspected, assessment by a liaison psychiatrist or other mental health professional is essential, considering that a diagnosis of personality disorder should not be made simply on the basis of behaviour during the current or previous admissions. Other factors, including pain, stress and abnormal glucose levels, may exacerbate personality traits (37). Strategies for managing patients with personality disorder are more likely to be successful if the patient, and if possible carers, are involved. Written contracts of care can be useful for maintaining focus on the fundamentals of care (38).

Assessment

All patients presenting to hospital with self-harm, suicidal behaviours or suicidal ideation should receive a full mental health assessment before discharge, ideally by a liaison psychiatry team well integrated with the treating medical (and diabetes) service. Patients with diabetes who are admitted with self-harm or a suicidal attempt should routinely be asked about suicidal ideation and whether they have considered using insulin as a means to attempt suicide by a member of the admitting team (39).

Assessing Suicidal Thoughts

Some authors have suggested that physicians involved in the care of people with diabetes should be able to ask about suicidal thoughts if necessary (17). Although many non-mental health professionals may be afraid of triggering such thoughts by asking about them, there is no evidence to suggest that asking about suicidal thoughts will do so (40). If anything, the evidence is that by asking about them, you are giving the person an opportunity to discuss them, and even this alone may be a relief. It is important to ask, and thus not to miss the presence of suicidal intent. Taking a gentle and sensitive approach is key. Remember that thoughts of self-harm or suicide may exist on a spectrum, from a passive death wish (a sense that if they were to die in their sleep this would not be unwelcome) to having suicidal thoughts, with or without an intention to act on them, and at the more extreme end there may be suicidal plans. Planning may include stockpiling medication or other means, writing notes, making a will and/or giving things away. Some people will have intrusive, unwelcome thoughts that they fear and have no wish to act upon. Some will have chronic thoughts of self-harm and may find that these come to the fore at times of stress.

It will feel more natural to introduce questioning around a cue given by the patients or to follow up on questions about mood by asking the following, for example: 'It sounds like you've really been struggling lately. Sometimes, when people are having a difficult time, they may feel like they cannot go on. Have you ever felt like this?' A positive answer is followed up with more questioning about intent and planning (41). Having thoughts of self-harm alone does not mean that the person is likely to act on them, but they will likely require a more in-depth assessment (42).

The American Diabetes Association recommends an assessment of mental health in patients with diabetes at their initial assessment and periodically thereafter, especially when there is a significant change in their illness, treatment or other relevant circumstances (43).

Diabetes distress, depression and suicidal ideation are not routinely assessed or screened for in patients with diabetes in Europe: NICE guidelines for DKA in children and young adults and for adults do not include psychological assessment or management after an episode of DKA. In the UK, the DKA guidelines of the Joint British Diabetes Societies (JBDS) recommend that psychological support is delivered by a member of the diabetes

Table 9.1 'Red flags' for formal psychiatric evaluation in diabetes.

Suicidal ideation or behaviours

Evidence of depressed mood

Recurrent admissions (i.e. for recurrent diabetic ketoacidosis or severe hypoglycaemia)

Difficulties at transition from paediatric to adult services

Persistent suboptimal glycaemic control

Low body mass index (may indicate eating disorder)

Reluctance to commence insulin therapy in type 2 diabetes (consider needle phobia)

Adapted from Garrett and Doherty (45).

team prior to discharge as an audit standard. The JBDS–Royal College of Psychiatrists (RCPsych) guidelines note that this is unlikely to be adequate to identify and manage significant psychiatric morbidity (23). They recommend that all patients who present with rDKA (which they define as two or more unexplained episodes of DKA) should have a formal mental health assessment, preferably by a liaison psychiatrist with expertise in diabetes. The JBDS–RCPsych guidelines acknowledge that patients with psychological and social problems may struggle to access the usual pathways and to access diabetes care. Using DKA as a red flag for a psychiatric assessment will improve detection of these problems.

Custal et al. suggested that patients with type 1 diabetes may not use self-harm in order to deal with emotions, as they may engage in insulin misuse instead. Where low levels of motivation to change and/or insulin abuse are suspected in type 1 diabetes patients, it may be helpful to consider the individual's personality and the role of insulin abuse when determining the appropriate intervention (44). Boileau et al. recommended that all children with more than two repeated comas within a three-month period should be admitted to hospital to allow for full evaluation and for multidisciplinary support once it has been discussed that secret self-administration of insulin is suspected (22).

Self-administration of insulin while in hospital should be carefully considered for people who definitely self-harm and may require supervision. It may be useful to have a 'red flag' system to identify patients who require referral for formal psychiatric assessment and treatment, as outlined in Table 9.1 (45).

Management

Although there are clear guidelines for the management of diabetes emergencies, there are few studies or guidelines that inform the management of patients with diabetes and mental illness where psychological considerations play an important role in the aetiology of ostensibly physical presentations. Yet the inpatient medical admission should be regarded as a 'window of opportunity' to identify the need for and initiate integrating psychological care in order to support self-management (23).

Restriction of Access to Lethal Means

There is international evidence that by restricting access to lethal means overall rates of death by suicide can be reduced (46). This was first noted with the reduction of the carbon monoxide content of coal gas in the UK in the 1960s effecting a reduction in suicide not only by this means, but by any means (47). When pack sizes of over-the-counter analgesic medications (including paracetamol) were reduced in the UK, there was a significant long-term reduction in the numbers of deaths due to hepatotoxicity secondary to paracetamol (48). It is impossible, however, to avoid insulin for patients with diabetes who need it. Consideration should be given for maximising supervision for people deemed to be high risk (e.g. those who have been admitted with overt or occult overdose of insulin).

Treatments

The psychiatric assessment will guide the treatment required. If a mood disorders is present, this should be treated so as to be consistent with best clinical practice. Similarly, if there is a psychotic illness, substance abuse disorder or personality disorder present, these conditions should be treated as the primary means of reducing suicidal risk into the future.

In the management of depression, NICE Clinical Guideline 91 addresses the treatment of depression in chronic physical health conditions, although not specifically diabetes (39). These guidelines adapt the stepped care model for depression, including psychological and social interventions and antidepressants. A key underlying principle is that of collaborative care, as integrating the treatment of depression with the optimisation of diabetes management, ideally within the same clinical team, is likely to lead to improved outcomes for both conditions than segregating their care (49).

Family therapy, out-of-hours diabetes support and active follow-up by diabetes educators as part of transition care teams (overseeing the transition from paediatric to adult services) have been shown to reduce the number of admissions in young people with type 1 diabetes (50, 51).

Other Harm-Related Issues

There may be other reasons why an individual might misuse their insulin or other hypoglycaemic agents, although these may be difficult to identify and manage. Specific mood changes caused by changes in blood glucose concentrations may be idiosyncratic, and although negative affective states are the most common, positive changes such as giddiness and euphoria are also seen. Boileau et al. were unable to identify a predictor of secret insulin self-injections (22). Some people report a 'hypoglycaemic rush', which may result in the abuse of hypoglycaemic agents (52). Cassidy et al. reported a case of a patient without any history of a psychiatric disorder who misused insulin regularly over a two-year period for its euphoric effects. His regular insulin misuse went unrecognised until he developed a depressive illness and presented with a serious suicide attempt. The authors recommended that all healthcare professionals should be alert to the possibility of insulin misuse and should consider psychological evaluation for patients with persistent poor glycaemic control in diabetes (53).

Patients with a dual diagnosis (with mental health and substance use problems) may have particular difficulty in managing both psychiatric and diabetic treatments due to the typical complex and chaotic behaviour associated with substance use. Additional medical complications such as infection risk and injection site risks with diabetes and the risk of developing additional physical disorders (e.g. liver disease) can make their management highly challenging. Factitious consideration may be present as well, and this may present difficulties in diagnosis, which must be made very carefully (25). Other forms of psychiatric comorbidity may present similar challenges (e.g. mental illness and developmental disorder, mental illness and personality disorder, etc.).

Conclusion

As mental disorders are common in diabetes and are also associated with attempted and completed suicide, it is important to be vigilant for these symptoms among people with diabetes. Having a system for ensuring the assessment of people who have 'red flags' for mental illness will be helpful in facilitating the early assessment and treatment of these important, life-threatening conditions. In particular, unexplained presentations with DKA or hypoglycaemia should trigger a detailed assessment.

References

1 WHO. *The ICD-10 Classification of Mental and Behavioural Disorders: Clinical Descriptions and Diagnostic Guidelines.* World Health Organization, 1992.

2 Robins E, Murphy GE, Wilkinson RH Jr, Gassner S, Kayes J. Some clinical considerations in the prevention of suicide based on a study of 134 successful suicides. *Am J Public Health Nations Health.* 1959; 49(7): 888–99.

3 Qin P. The impact of psychiatric illness on suicide: differences by diagnosis of disorders and by sex and age of subjects. *J Psychiatr Res.* 2011; 45(11): 1445–52.

4 Shahtahmasebi S. Suicides by mentally ill people. *ScientificWorldJournal.* 2003; 3: 684–93.

5 Bowers L, Banda T, Nijman H. Suicide inside: a systematic review of inpatient suicides. *J Nerv Ment Dis.* 2010; 198(5): 315–28.

6 Srivastava A. Psychological attributes and socio-demographic profile of hundred completed suicide victims in the state of Goa, India. *Indian J Psychiatry.* 2013; 55(3): 268–72.

7 Parra Uribe I, Blasco-Fontecilla H, Garcia-Pares G, Giro Batalla M, Llorens Capdevila M, Cebria Meca A, et al. Attempted and completed suicide: not what we expected? *J Affect Disord.* 2013; 150(3): 840–6.

8 Giner L, Blasco-Fontecilla H, Mercedes Perez-Rodriguez M, Garcia-Nieto R, Giner J, Guija JA, et al. Personality disorders and health problems distinguish suicide attempters from completers in a direct comparison. *J Affect Disord.* 2013; 151(2): 474–83.

9 Mohan C, Tembo V, McNicholas B, Doherty AM. Defining high risk by clinical lethality: the different characteristics and management of the survivors of serious self-injury admitted to critical care, compared with lower lethality self-injury. *Gen Hosp Psychiatry.* 2020; 64: 131–2.

10 Snoek FJ, Pouwer F, Welch GW, Polonsky WH. Diabetes-related emotional distress in Dutch and U.S. diabetic patients: cross-cultural validity of the problem areas in diabetes scale. *Diabetes Care.* 2000; 23(9): 1305–9.

11 NICE. *Self-Harm. Quality Standard [QS34].* National Institute for Health and Care Excellence, 2013.

12 Doshi A, Boudreaux ED, Wang N, Pelletier AJ, Camargo CA Jr. National study of US emergency department visits for attempted suicide and self-inflicted injury, 1997–2001. *Ann Emerg Med.* 2005; 46(4): 369–75.

13 Fegan J, Doherty AM. Adjustment disorder and suicidal behaviours presenting in the general medical setting: a systematic review. *Int J Environ Res Public Health.* 2019; 16(16): 2967.

14 Roberts SE, Goldacre MJ, Neil HA. Mortality in young people admitted to hospital for diabetes: database study. *BMJ.* 2004; 328(7442): 741–2.

15 Roy A, Roy M, Janal M. Suicide attempts and ideation in African-American type 1 diabetic patients. *Psychiatry Res.* 2010; 179(1): 53–6.

16 Lofman S, Hakko H, Mainio A, Timonen M, Rasanen P. Characteristics of suicide among diabetes patients: a population based study of suicide victims in northern Finland. *J Psychosom Res*. 2012; 73(4): 268–71.

17 Pompili M, Forte A, Lester D, Erbuto D, Rovedi F, Innamorati M, et al. Suicide risk in type 1 diabetes mellitus: a systematic review. *J Psychosom Res*. 2014; 76(5): 352–60.

18 Petit JM, Goueslard K, Chauvet-Gelinier JC, Bouillet B, Vergès B, Jollant F, Quantin C. Association between hospital admission for ketoacidosis and subsequent suicide attempt in young adults with type 1 diabetes. *Diabetologia*. 2020; 63: 1745–52.

19 Russell KS, Stevens JR, Stern TA. Insulin overdose among patients with diabetes: a readily available means of suicide. *Prim Care Companion J Clin Psychiatry*. 2009; 11 (5): 258–62.

20 von Mach MA, Meyer S, Omogbehin B, Kann PH, Weilemann LS. Epidemiological assessment of 160 cases of insulin overdose recorded in a regional poisons unit. *Int J Clin Pharmacol Ther*. 2004; 42 (5): 277–80.

21 Kjaerulff M, Astrup BS. Sudden death due to diabetic ketoacidosis following power failure of an insulin pump: autopsy and pump data. *J Forensic Leg Med*. 2019; 63: 34–9.

22 Boileau P, Aboumrad B, Bougneres P. Recurrent comas due to secret self-administration of insulin in adolescents with type 1 diabetes. *Diabetes Care*. 2006; 29(2): 430–1.

23 JBDS, RCPsych. *The Management of Diabetes in Adults and Children with Psychiatric Disorders in Inpatient Settings.* Joint British Diabetes Societies and Royal College of Psychiatrists, 2017.

24 Umpierrez G, Korytkowski M. Diabetic emergencies – ketoacidosis, hyperglycaemic hyperosmolar state and hypoglycaemia. *Nat Rev Endocrinol*. 2016; 12(4): 222–32.

25 Williams G. What goes around, comes around. *Lancet*. 2012; 379(9833): 2235–6.

26 Bryden KS, Dunger DB, Mayou RA, Peveler RC, Neil HA. Poor prognosis of young adults with type 1 diabetes: a longitudinal study. *Diabetes Care*. 2003; 26 (4): 1052–7.

27 Pelizza L, Pupo S. Brittle diabetes: psychopathology and personality. *J Diabetes Complications*. 2016; 30(8): 1544–7.

28 Garrett CJ, Choudhary P, Amiel SA, Fonagy P, Ismail K. Recurrent diabetic ketoacidosis and a brief history of brittle diabetes research: contemporary and past evidence in diabetic ketoacidosis research including mortality, mental health and prevention. *Diabet Med*. 2019; 36(11): 1329–35.

29 Goldston DB, Kelley AE, Reboussin DM, Daniel SS, Smith JA, Schwartz RP, et al. Suicidal ideation and behavior and noncompliance with the medical regimen among diabetic adolescents. *J Am Acad Child Adolesc Psychiatry*. 1997; 36(11): 1528–36.

30 Binks CA, Fenton M, McCarthy L, Lee T, Adams CE, Duggan C. Psychological therapies for people with borderline personality disorder. *Cochrane Database Syst Rev*. 2006; (1): CD005652.

31 Oldham JM. Borderline personality disorder and suicidality. *Am J Psychiatry*. 2006; 163(1): 20–6.

32 Leichsenring F, Leibing E, Kruse J, New AS, Leweke F. Borderline personality disorder. *Lancet*. 2011; 377(9759): 74–84.

33 Attwood J, Wilkinson-Tough M, Lambe S, Draper E. Improving attitudes towards personality disorder: is training for health and social care professionals effective? *J Pers Disord*. 2019: 1–23.

34 Holmqvist R. Staff feelings and patient diagnosis. *Can J Psychiatry*. 2000; 45(4): 349–56.

35 Tyrer P. Why we need to take personality disorder out of the doghouse. *Br J Psychiatry*. 2020; 216(2): 65–6.

36 Cristea IA, Gentili C, Cotet CD, Palomba D, Barbui C, Cuijpers P. Efficacy of psychotherapies for borderline personality disorder: a systematic review and meta-

analysis. *JAMA Psychiatry*. 2017; 74(4): 319–28.

37 Krahn DD, Mackenzie TB. Organic personality syndrome caused by insulin-related nocturnal hypoglycemia. *Psychosomatics*. 1984; 25(9): 711–2.

38 McEnany GW, Tescher BE. Contracting for care. One nursing approach to the hospitalized borderline patient. *J Psychosoc Nurs Ment Health Serv*. 1985; 23(4): 11–8.

39 NICE. *Depression: The Treatment and Management of Depression in Adults (Clinical Guideline 90)*. National Institute of Health and Care Excellence, 2009.

40 Dazzi T, Gribble R, Wessely S, Fear NT. Does asking about suicide and related behaviours induce suicidal ideation? What is the evidence? *Psychol Med*. 2014; 44(16): 3361–3.

41 O'Reilly M, Kiyimba N, Karim K. 'This is a question we have to ask everyone': asking young people about self-harm and suicide. *J Psychiatr Ment Health Nurs*. 2016; 23(8): 479–88.

42 Mars B, Heron J, Klonsky ED, Moran P, O'Connor RC, Tilling K, et al. Predictors of future suicide attempt among adolescents with suicidal thoughts or non-suicidal self-harm: a population-based birth cohort study. *Lancet Psychiatry*. 2019; 6(4): 327–37.

43 Young-Hyman D, de Groot M, Hill-Briggs F, Gonzalez JS, Hood K, Peyrot M. Psychosocial care for people with diabetes: a position statement of the American Diabetes Association. *Diabetes Care*. 2016; 39(12): 2126–40.

44 Custal N, Arcelus J, Aguera Z, Bove FI, Wales J, Granero R, et al. Treatment outcome of patients with comorbid type 1 diabetes and eating disorders. *BMC Psychiatry*. 2014; 14: 140.

45 Garrett C, Doherty A. Diabetes and mental health. *Clin Med (Lond)*. 2014; 14(6): 669–72.

46 Nordentoft M, Qin P, Helweg-Larsen K, Juel K. Restrictions in means for suicide: an effective tool in preventing suicide: the Danish experience. *Suicide Life Threat Behav*. 2007; 37(6): 688–97.

47 Kreitman N. The coal gas story. United Kingdom suicide rates, 1960–71. *Br J Prev Soc Med*. 1976; 30(2): 86–93.

48 Hawton K, Simkin S, Deeks J, Cooper J, Johnston A, Waters K, et al. UK legislation on analgesic packs: before and after study of long term effect on poisonings. *BMJ*. 2004; 329(7474): 1076.

49 Katon WJ, Lin EH, Von Korff M, Ciechanowski P, Ludman EJ, Young B, et al. Collaborative care for patients with depression and chronic illnesses. *N Engl J Med*. 2010; 363(27): 2611–20.

50 Ellis DA, Frey MA, Naar-King S, Templin T, Cunningham P, Cakan N. Use of multisystemic therapy to improve regimen adherence among adolescents with type 1 diabetes in chronic poor metabolic control: a randomized controlled trial. *Diabetes Care*. 2005; 28(7): 1604–10.

51 Holmes-Walker DJ, Llewellyn AC, Farrell K. A transition care programme which improves diabetes control and reduces hospital admission rates in young adults with type 1 diabetes aged 15–25 years. *Diabet Med*. 2007; 24(7): 764–9.

52 Wazaify M, Abushams L, Van Hout MC. Abuse of sulfonylureas: is factitious hypoglycemia a cause for concern? *Int J Clin Pharm*. 2019; 41(1): 3–5.

53 Cassidy EM, O'Halloran DJ, Barry S. Insulin as a substance of misuse in a patient with insulin dependent diabetes mellitus. *BMJ*. 1999; 319(7222): 1417–8.

Chapter 1

Obesity and Mental Health

Aoife M. Egan

Introduction

Over 650 million people live with obesity worldwide, and almost all countries are affected by what is considered a global obesity pandemic (1). Body mass index (BMI) is a crude population measure of obesity, but it is commonly used in clinical practice as it is cheap and convenient. It is calculated by dividing a person's weight (in kilograms) by the square of their height (in metres). A person with a BMI of $\geq 30 \text{ kg/m}^2$ is considered obese (1). Obesity is associated with an increased risk of multiple adverse health complications, including cardiovascular disease, diabetes and cancer (2). It is also one of the factors that contribute to excess premature mortality in patients with severe mental illness (SMI), who die 15–20 years younger than the general population (3). There is evidence that this mortality gap is widening rather than closing (4). Mental health disorders are also highly prevalent worldwide, and the World Health Organization (WHO) estimates that one in four people will be affected at some point in their lives (5).

It is therefore not unexpected that obesity and mental health disorders frequently co-occur (Figure 10.1); however, as outlined in the following section, there is a large body of evidence suggesting a bidirectional relationship between obesity and a variety of mental health disorders.

Obesity and Mood Disorders

A systematic review and meta-analysis of studies examining the longitudinal, bidirectional relationship between depression and obesity found that obesity at baseline increased the risk of onset of depression at follow-up (odds ratio (OR) = 1.55; 95% confidence interval (CI) = 1.22–1.98). However, depression also increased the odds for developing obesity (OR = 1.58; 95% CI= 1.33–1.87) (6). Indeed, depressive symptoms in adolescence appear to predict elevated BMI in adulthood (7). Additional data reveal that almost 50% of patients with bipolar disorder are obese – a proportion that is well above that of the general population (8).

Considering the symptoms associated with mood disorders, including poor energy, sleep disturbance and decreased motivation, it is not surprising that most studies document weight increases in affected populations over time (9, 10). There is an extensive body of research attempting to tease out the biological mechanisms underpinning the association between mood disorders and obesity. Disturbances in cortisol are common in people with depression. This may be due to poor sleep affecting the usual circadian production of this hormone. The described clinical changes are similar, albeit milder, to those that occur in Cushing's syndrome (Chapter 5), such as visceral weight gain (11). Additional hormones linked to weight regulation, including leptin and adiponectin, are also altered in mood

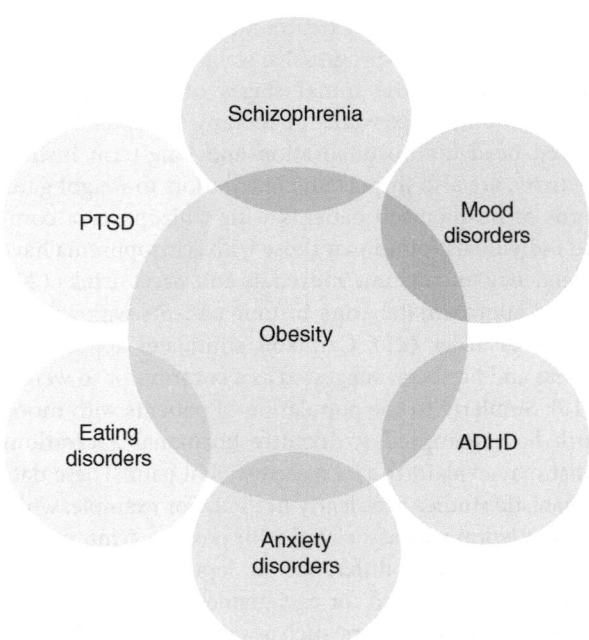

Figure 10.1 Overlap between obesity and mental health disorders. ADHD: attention-deficit hyperactivity disorder; PTSD: post-traumatic stress disorder.

disorders and may contribute to the development of obesity in this population (10). Furthermore, it is increasingly recognised that both obesity and mood disorders are associated with chronic low-grade inflammation, a factor that could potentially fuel the relationship between the two conditions (12). Finally, the role of pharmacotherapy must not be overlooked when examining the topic of depression and subsequent obesity risk. Many of the agents used to treat depression are associated with sedation and increased appetite, with consequent weight gain (Chapter 3) (13).

Looking at the relationship in reverse, it is well established that people with obesity feel stigmatised and experience discrimination in education, employment and healthcare (14). This experience, along with associated physical limitations, pain and burden of comorbidities, could understandably trigger depressive symptoms. People with extreme obesity are almost five times more likely to have experienced an episode of major depression in the past year compared to their average-weight counterparts (15). Interestingly, weight stigma appears to affect women disproportionately, making them more vulnerable to a variety of mental health disorders compared to men (16). Further studies are necessary to clarify additional risk factors for the development of mood disorders among people with obesity.

Obesity and Schizophrenia

Schizophrenia is a mental illness associated with long-term disability and has a prevalence of approximately 1% worldwide (17). Its symptoms include psychosis, apathy, withdrawal and cognitive impairment, and it is associated with numerous physical diseases, including diabetes and cardiovascular disease (9). Before the onset of the illness, future schizophrenia patients do not weigh more than their peers, but as the illness progresses, 50% become obese (18). Antipsychotic medications are the mainstay of treatment in confirmed schizophrenia, and they undoubtedly play a large role in the progressive weight gain observed in this population. This is particularly observed in the initial stages of treatment, with significant weight gain occurring even in the first six weeks of therapy (Chapter 3) (19). Lifestyle factors, including the increased need for hospitalisation and long-term institutional care with lower levels of daily activity, are also important contributors to weight gain. A study examining the dietary patterns of hospitalised patients with schizophrenia compared to healthy age- and sex-matched individuals found that those with schizophrenia have poor nutritional patterns and have a tendency to consume more fats and sweet drinks (20). A meta-analysis of 35 studies found that approximately one in four patients with schizophrenia had a diagnosis of cannabis use disorder (21). Cannabis stimulates appetite via activation of the endocannabinoid system and has been suggested as a contributor to weight gain in patients with schizophrenia (10). Similarly to the population of patients with mood disorders, a significant body of work has attempted to identify hormonal aberrations among patients with schizophrenia that may explain the increased weight gain. These data are often conflicting, and further mechanistic studies are clearly needed. For example, while one study found that an increase in serum leptin was associated with positive symptoms in patients with schizophrenia, there was no overall difference in leptin concentrations between those with schizophrenia and controls matched for age, gender and ethnicity at a group level (22). Leptin can also be influenced by factors such as age, gender, BMI and antipsychotic medications, making the interpretation of population-based studies challenging (23, 24).

Obesity and Attention-Deficit Hyperactivity Disorder

Attention-deficit hyperactivity disorder (ADHD) has a prevalence of over 5% in school-aged children and persists into adulthood in up to 65% of cases (25, 26). It is characterised by an age-inappropriate and impairing pattern of inattention and/or hyperactivity/impulsivity (27). A systematic review of 42 studies including 728,136 individuals noted a significant association between obesity and ADHD in both children (OR 1.2 = 95% CI = 1.05–1.37) and adults (OR = 1.55, 95% CI = 1.32–1.81) (28). A number of studies have suggested that decreased physical activity from a younger age may promote weight gain in these individuals (29, 30). In addition, people with ADHD find it difficult to organise meals and often eat impulsively (10). Of interest is a study that suggested that the obesity-related *FTO* gene modulated the risk for ADHD, and another study identified common obesity risk alleles in childhood ADHD, suggesting a common genetic background in ADHD and obesity (31, 32). Additional work suggests that genetically determined dysfunctions in the dopaminergic system in people with obesity and ADHD result in an increase in reward-seeking behaviours, including increased food consumption (9).

Obesity and Eating Disorders

While disordered eating (including night-time eating) is common among people with obesity, binge-eating disorder is the most frequently diagnosed eating disorder in obesity (14). An episode of binge eating is characterised by eating in a discrete period of time, such as a two-hour period, an amount of food that is larger than most people would eat in a similar period of time. People have a sense of a lack of control over the eating and often feel uncomfortably full, disgusted or guilty after overeating. People with binge-eating disorder experience episodes at least once per week (33). Binge-eating disorder occurs in up to 30% of obese individuals and is more prevalent among those who are severely obese and those seeking obesity treatments (34, 35). The restraint model hypothesises that binge eating originates from shape and weight concerns that lead to repetitive patterns of dietary restraint followed by binge eating (36). Alternatively, the affect regulation model suggests that binge eating is a coping mechanism to reduce negative feelings, and the escape theory describes binge eating as a strategy that allows the person to focus on the stimulus at hand and avoid self-awareness and other stressors (36, 37). Smaller percentages of patients with obesity have bulimia nervosa, where the binge eating is accompanied by self-induced vomiting or other behaviours such as excessive exercise or misuse of laxatives (14).

In addition to the aforementioned conditions, people with obesity appear to be at increased risk of substance abuse and anxiety disorders (14). In recent years, post-traumatic stress disorder has also emerged as a risk factor for the development of obesity (9).

Psychiatric Evaluation of Obese Patients

Overall, it is clear that obesity is associated with a significant psychological burden, and people with obesity are vulnerable from a mental health viewpoint. When possible, we recommend formal psychosocial evaluation of patients with obesity. This is particularly important in those who are seeking obesity treatment. Modern obesity management takes a multidisciplinary approach to care, and ideally patients will have access to mental health professionals who can perform detailed evaluations. The format of these evaluations varies, but they typically take the form of clinical interviews combined with validated question-naires to evaluate psychiatric symptoms (38). It is particularly important to enquire about problematic eating patterns, weight control practices and loss of control related to eating (39). Major psychiatric illness and substance abuse disorders should be identified. A bespoke plan can be developed to address mental health issues that arise during the evaluation. This may include lifestyle modification counselling, supportive psychotherapy or psychotropic medications (14). When choosing psychotropic medications in this popu-lation, careful consideration should be given to agents that are less likely to promote weight gain (Chapter 3).

In recognising the importance of treating mental health disorders, most bariatric surgery programmes now insist on mental health evaluation prior to progressing with an invasive weight-loss intervention (40). This allows for identification of potential post-operative challenges (e.g. binge-eating behaviours) and facilitates behavioural change to support long-term weight loss. Active substance abuse, bulimia nervosa and poorly con-trolled depression are generally considered contraindications to bariatric surgery (14). The assessment should include an exploration of the person's reasons for seeking surgery at this time. In order for this to be successful, it is important that the patient is seeking surgery for reasons that are consistent with a reasonable expectation of the outcome (41). Such reasons may include reduced weight and improved health across parameters including improved mobility, reduced cardiovascular risk, improved energy levels, etc. However, when patients are seeking surgery due to external/peer pressure the likelihood of success is much reduced, as is the case when they are unduly influenced by body-image considerations. Their expectations following surgery must be similarly realistic: people who expect a cathartic life change and the resolution of all their current problems are likely to develop difficulties with post-operative compliance and are at higher risk of developing mood disorders (42).

The Effects of Weight Loss on Mental Health

Mainstream treatments for weight loss include lifestyle interventions, pharmacotherapy and bariatric surgery. At 6–12 months, these options are associated with approximate mean weight losses of 5–8%, 5–10% and 15–30%, respectively (43). The sleeve gastrectomy and Roux-en-Y gastric bypass are now the most commonly performed bariatric surgeries. The laparoscopic adjustable gastric band has fallen out of favour due to poorer clinical outcomes, and the biliopancreatic diversion is rarely performed. Endoscopic weight-loss procedures such as intra-gastric balloons and the endoscopic sleeve gastroplasty are also gaining popularity, but there is less evidence to support their efficacy. Available and approved weight-loss medications vary worldwide. When prescribing these medications, one should bear in mind their mechanism of action, possible side effects and potential interactions with psychotropic medications. For example, phenteramine, the most widely prescribed weight-loss medication in the USA, is a norepinephrine-releasing agent and is contraindicated in the setting of monoamine oxidase inhibitors (43).

In general, moderate weight loss consisting of a 5–10% reduction in baseline weight is associated with clinical improvements in obesity-related disorders and metabolic risk factors such as blood pressure and lipid profiles (43). Larger weight loss, as seen with bariatric surgery, can be associated with even more dramatic improvements in physical health, such as remission of type 2 diabetes (44). Effects of weight loss on mental health outcomes have also been evaluated in a number of studies.

The psychological changes following weight loss as a result of behavioural and/or dietary weight-loss interventions were evaluated in a 2014 systematic review of 36 studies (45). Changes in self-esteem, depressive symptoms, body image and health-related quality of life were evaluated. In the setting of an intervention, there were consistent improvements in these psychological outcomes concurrent with, but sometimes even without, weight loss. However, lifestyle interventions tend to be very heterogeneous in design, and this was reflected in the considerable variation in effect size noted. In addition, only nine of the studies included a suitable control group. Overall, however, the larger body of evidence would suggest that, in general, weight loss is associated with improvements in psychosocial status, including health- and weight-related quality of life, self-esteem and sexual functioning (14, 46). The improvements are more marked in people who undergo bariatric surgery, suggesting that the response is linked to the magnitude of weight loss (14).

The interactions between weight loss and formal psychopathology are less clear, and most relevant studies have focused on patients undergoing bariatric surgery. There appears to be a particularly high prevalence (over 50%) of mental health disorders among this group at the time of presentation for surgical evaluation, particularly mood and anxiety disorders (40, 47). It is also important to be aware that approximately one in three female patients undergoing bariatric surgery have experienced childhood sexual abuse (48). This appears to be a risk factor for psychiatric hospitalisation after bariatric surgery and may impact poorly on post-surgical weight loss (46). It has been hypothesised that in cases where the individual has suffered sexual assault in childhood, or indeed adulthood, weight gain may have served a function in avoiding unwanted sexual attention, and that the removal of this defence leaves the individual feeling suddenly unprotected and vulnerable (49). Interestingly, a US cohort study in which 57% of patients undergoing bariatric surgery had a preoperative mental illness (44% mild to moderate depression or anxiety, 6% severe depression or anxiety, 6% bipolar, psychotic or schizophrenia spectrum disorder) found that there were no differences in weight loss among patients with mental illness or patients taking psychiatric medications after up to seven years of follow-up (47). A 2016 systematic review and meta-analysis of 27 publications reported that associations between preoperative mental health conditions and weight-loss outcomes post-bariatric surgery were conflicting. However, bariatric surgery was consistently associated with post-operative decreases in the prevalence of depression (seven studies; 8–74% decrease) and the severity of depressive symptoms (six studies; 40–70% decrease) (50). The increase in physical activity observed in post-bariatric surgery patients may contribute to these positive changes (46).

Despite an improvement in the prevalence of depression, multiple studies have found an increased rate of suicide among people who have undergone bariatric surgery (46). This is exemplified by a 2018 publication by Neovius et al. (51). The study included patients from the prospective Swedish Obese Subjects (SOS) study, which compared bariatric surgery with usual obesity care, and from the Scandinavian Obesity Surgery Registry (SOReg), which included patients who had gastric bypass matched to individuals treated with intensive lifestyle modification (51). In both the SOS and the SOReg surgical groups, suicides or non-fatal self-harm events were higher than in the non-surgical comparisons (adjusted hazard ratios = 1.78 (95% CI = 1.23–2.57, p = 0.0021) and 3.16 (95% CI = 2.46–4.06), respectively). Another registry study based in Sweden noted that the increased risk of post-surgery self-harm and hospitalisation for depression mainly occurs in patients who have a pre-surgical diagnosis of self-harm or depression. This again highlights the importance of a thorough, preoperative psychological evaluation to identify at-risk individuals (52).

There is also evidence that some individuals develop substance abuse issues after bariatric surgery. King et al. noted that the prevalence of alcohol use disorder symptoms did not significantly differ from one year before to one year after bariatric surgery (7.6% versus 7.3%, p = 0.98), but significantly increased in the second post-operative year (9.6%, p = 0.01) (53). People who had a history of alcohol use disorder and those who had regular alcohol consumption (two or more alcoholic drinks per week) were at greater risk. Undergoing Roux-en-Y gastric bypass versus laparoscopic adjustable gastric banding is associated with double the risk of alcohol use disorder symptoms (54). We await data on the incidence of alcohol use disorder symptoms after sleeve gastrectomy. Animal studies suggest a neurobiological basis for increased alcohol reward following Roux-en-Y gastric bypass surgery, and pharmacokinetic studies have shown increased peak blood alcohol concentrations following this surgery (55). Similarly, use of illicit drugs (predominantly marijuana) appears to increase after Roux-en-Y gastric bypass (54). In light of these data, certain bariatric surgery programmes recommend the avoidance of any alcohol intake following bariatric surgery. The concept of 'addiction transfer' has been commonly used in this context. This theory suggests that patients undergoing bariatric surgery may replace a food addiction with an alternative addiction. The theory has not been clinically validated, but available evidence points towards the importance of post-operative screening for substance-related problems in the bariatric surgery population (56).

Finally, it is important to be aware that malabsorptive bariatric procedures such as the Roux-en-Y gastric bypass or biliopancreatic diversion may result in significant changes to medication pharmacodynamics and pharmacokinetics. In practice, drugs are typically converted to immediate-release forms where possible. However, it is not clear whether this is effective, and close monitoring of symptoms (with plasma levels if appropriate) in patients receiving psychotropic drugs is recommended (46).

Conclusion

Both obesity and mental health disorders are highly prevalent and frequently occur in the same individual. While weight loss is typically associated with improvements in psychological functioning, a certain proportion of patients will develop new psychological issues or experience a relapse of pre-existing conditions. Further work is needed to clarify the underlying biological mechanisms explaining the relationship between obesity and mental health. In the interim, people with obesity should receive care in a multidisciplinary setting with access to mental health professionals who can address their individual psychological needs.

References

1   World Health Organization. Obesity. Available from: www.who.int/topics/obesity/en

2   Afshin A, Forouzanfar MH, Reitsma MB, Sur P, Estep K, Lee A, et al. Health effects of overweight and obesity in 195 countries over 25 years. *N Engl J Med*. 2017; 377(1): 13–27.

3   Wahlbeck K, Westman J, Nordentoft M, Gissler M, Laursen TM. Outcomes of Nordic mental health systems: life expectancy of patients with mental disorders. *Br J Psychiatry*. 2011; 199(6): 453–8.

4   Barber S, Thornicroft G. Reducing the mortality gap in people with severe mental disorders: the role of lifestyle psychosocial interventions. *Front Psychiatry*. 2018; 9: 463.

5   World Health Organization. The World Health Report 2001: Mental disorders affect one in four people, 2001. Available from: www.who.int/whr/2001/media_centre/press_release/en

6   Luppino FS, de Wit LM, Bouvy PF, Stijnen T, Cuijpers P, Penninx BWJH, Zitman FG. Overweight, obesity, and depression: a systematic review and meta-analysis of longitudinal studies. *Arch Gen Psychiatry*. 2010; 67(3): 220–9.

7   Franko DL, Striegel-Moore RH, Thompson D, Schreiber GB, Daniels SR. Does adolescent depression predict obesity in black and white young adult women? *Psychol Med*. 2005; 35(10): 1505–13.

8   Fiedorowicz JG, Palagummi NM, Forman-Hoffman VL, Miller DD, Haynes WG. Elevated prevalence of obesity, metabolic syndrome, and cardiovascular risk factors in bipolar disorder. *Ann Clin Psychiatry*. 2008; 20(3): 131–7.

9   Avila C, Holloway AC, Hahn MK, Morrison KM, Restivo M, Anglin R, Taylor VH. An overview of links between obesity and mental health. *Curr Obes Rep*. 2015; 4 (3): 303–10.

10 Taylor VH, McIntyre RS, Remington G, Levitan RD, Stonehocker B, Sharma AM. Beyond pharmacotherapy: understanding the links between obesity and chronic mental illness. *Can J Psychiatry*. 2012; 57 (1): 5–12.

11 Brown ES, Varghese FP, McEwen BS. Association of depression with medical illness: does cortisol play a role? *Biol Psychiatry*. 2004; 55(1): 1–9.

12 Shelton RC, Miller AH. Inflammation in depression: is adiposity a cause? *Dialogues Clin Neurosci*. 2011; 13(1): 41–53.

13 Kemp DE. Managing the side effects associated with commonly used treatments for bipolar depression. *J Affect Disord*. 2014; 169(Suppl. 1): S34–44.

14 Sarwer DB, Polonsky HM. The psychosocial burden of obesity. *Endocrinol Metab Clin North Am*. 2016; 45 (3): 677–88.

15 Onyike CU, Crum RM, Lee HB, Lyketsos CG, Eaton WW. Is obesity associated with major depression? Results from the Third National Health and Nutrition Examination Survey. *Am J Epidemiol*. 2003; 158(12): 1139–47.

16 Tronieri JS, Wurst CM, Pearl RL, Allison KC. Sex differences in obesity and mental health. *Curr Psychiatry Rep*. 2017; 19(6): 29.

17 Mueser KT, McGurk SR. Schizophrenia. *Lancet*. 2004; 363(9426): 2063–72.

18 Britvic D, Maric NP, Doknic M, Pekic S, Andric S, Jasovic-Gasic M, Popovic V. Metabolic issues in psychotic disorders with the focus on first-episode patients: a review. *Psychiatr Danub*. 2013; 25(4): 410–5.

19 Zipursky RB, Gu H, Green AI, Perkins DO, Tohen MF, McEvoy JP, et al. Course and predictors of weight gain in people with first-episode psychosis treated with olanzapine or haloperidol. *Br J Psychiatry*. 2005; 187: 537–43.

20 Amani R. Is dietary pattern of schizophrenia patients different from healthy subjects? *BMC Psychiatry*. 2007; 7: 15.

21 Koskinen J, Löhönen J, Koponen H, Isohanni M, Miettunen J. Rate of cannabis use disorders in clinical samples of patients with schizophrenia: a meta-analysis. *Schizophr Bull*. 2010; 36(6): 1115–30.

22 Nurjono M, Neelamekam S, Lee J. Serum leptin and its relationship with psychopathology in schizophrenia. *Psychoneuroendocrinology*. 2014; 50: 149–54.

23 Sentissi O, Epelbaum J, Olié J-P, Poirier M-F. Leptin and ghrelin levels in patients with schizophrenia during different antipsychotics treatment: a review. *Schizophr Bull*. 2008; 34(6): 1189–99.

24 Al-Harithy RN. Relationship of leptin concentration to gender, body mass index and age in Saudi adults. *Saudi Med J*. 2004; 25(8): 1086–90.

25 Polanczyk G, de Lima MS, Horta BL, Biederman J, Rohde LA. The worldwide prevalence of ADHD: a systematic review and metaregression analysis. *Am J Psychiatry*. 2007; 164(6): 942–8.

26 Faraone SV, Biederman J, Mick E. The age-dependent decline of attention deficit hyperactivity disorder: a meta-analysis of follow-up studies. *Psychol Med*. 2006; 36(2): 159–65.

27 Moreira-Maia CR, Massuti R, Tessari L, Campani F, Akutagava-Martins GC, Cortese S, Rohde LA. Are ADHD medications under or over prescribed worldwide?: Protocol for a systematic review and meta-analysis. *Medicine (Baltimore)*. 2018; 97(24): e10923.

28 Cortese S, Moreira-Maia CR, St Fleur D, Morcillo-Peñalver C, Rohde LA, Faraone SV. Association between ADHD and obesity: a systematic review and meta-analysis. *Am J Psychiatry*. 2016; 173(1): 34–43.

29 Khalife N, Kantomaa M, Glover V, Tammelin T, Laitinen J, Ebeling H, et al. Childhood attention-deficit/hyperactivity disorder symptoms are risk factors for obesity and physical inactivity in adolescence. *J Am Acad Child Adolesc Psychiatry*. 2014; 53(4): 425–36.

30 Cortese S, Tessari L. Attention-deficit/hyperactivity disorder (ADHD) and obesity: update 2016. *Curr Psychiatry Rep*. 2017; 19(1): 4.

31 Albayrak Ö, Pütter C, Volckmar A-L, Cichon S, Hoffmann P, Nöthen MM, et al. Common obesity risk alleles in childhood attention-deficit/hyperactivity disorder. *Am J Med Genet B Neuropsychiatr Genet*. 2013; 162B(4): 295–305.

32 Choudhry Z, Sengupta SM, Grizenko N, Thakur GA, Fortier M-E, Schmitz N, Joober R. Association between obesity-related gene *FTO* and ADHD. *Obesity (Silver Spring)*. 2013; 21(12): E738–44.

33 Berkman N, Brownley K, Peat CEA. *Management and Outcomes of Binge-Eating Disorder*. Agency for Healthcare Research and Quality, 2015.

34 Brownley KA, Berkman ND, Peat CM, Lohr KN, Cullen KE, Bann CM, Bulik CM. Binge-eating disorder in adults: a systematic review and meta-analysis. *Ann Intern Med*. 2016; 165(6): 409–20.

35 Bruce B, Wilfley D. Binge eating among the overweight population: a serious and prevalent problem. *J Am Diet Assoc*. 1996; 96(1): 58–61.

36 McCuen-Wurst C, Ruggieri M, Allison KC. Disordered eating and obesity: associations

between binge-eating disorder, night-eating syndrome, and weight-related comorbidities. *Ann N Y Acad Sci.* 2018; 1411(1): 96–105.

37 Haedt-Matt AA, Keel PK. Revisiting the affect regulation model of binge eating: a meta-analysis of studies using ecological momentary assessment. *Psychol Bull.* 2011; 137(4): 660–81.

38 Pearl RL, Allison KC, Tronieri JS, Wadden TA. Reconsidering the psychosocial–behavioral evaluation required prior to bariatric surgery. *Obesity (Silver Spring).* 2018; 26(2): 249–50.

39 Devlin MJ, Yanovski SZ, Wilson GT. Obesity: what mental health professionals need to know. *Am J Psychiatry.* 2000; 157 (6): 854–66.

40 Sarwer DB, Wadden TA, Fabricatore AN. Psychosocial and behavioral aspects of bariatric surgery. *Obes Res.* 2005; 13(4): 639–48.

41 Bauchowitz A, Azarbad L, Day K, Gonder-Frederick L. Evaluation of expectations and knowledge in bariatric surgery patients. *Surg Obes Relat Dis.* 2007; 3(5): 554–8.

42 Walfish S, Vance D, Fabricatore AN. Psychological evaluation of bariatric surgery applicants: procedures and reasons for delay or denial of surgery. *Obes Surg.* 2007; 17(12): 1578–83.

43 Heymsfield SB, Wadden TA. Mechanisms, pathophysiology, and management of obesity. *N Engl J Med.* 2017; 376(15): 1492.

44 Jensen MD, Ryan DH, Apovian CM, Ard JD, Comuzzie AG, Donato KA, et al. 2013 AHA/ACC/TOS guideline for the management of overweight and obesity in adults: a report of the American College of Cardiology/American Heart Association Task Force on Practice Guidelines and The Obesity Society. *J Am Coll Cardiol.* 2014; 63 (25 Pt B): 2985–3023.

45 Lasikiewicz N, Myrissa K, Hoyland A, Lawton CL. Psychological benefits of weight loss following behavioural and/or dietary weight loss interventions.

A systematic research review. *Appetite.* 2014; 72: 123–37.

46 Morledge MD, Pories WJ. Mental health in bariatric surgery: selection, access, and outcomes. *Obesity (Silver Spring).* 2020; 28 (4): 689–95.

47 Fisher D, Coleman KJ, Arterburn DE, Fischer H, Yamamoto A, Young DR, et al. Mental illness in bariatric surgery: a cohort study from the PORTAL network. *Obesity (Silver Spring).* 2017; 25(5): 850–6.

48 Orcutt M, King WC, Kalarchian MA, Devlin MJ, Marcus MD, Garcia L, et al. The relationship between childhood maltreatment and psychopathology in adults undergoing bariatric surgery. *Surg Obes Relat Dis.* 2019; 15(2): 295–303.

49 Faden J, Leonard D, O'Reardon J, Hanson R. Obesity as a defense mechanism. *Int J Surg Case Rep.* 2013; 4(1): 127–9.

50 Dawes AJ, Maggard-Gibbons M, Maher AR, Booth MJ, Miake-Lye I, Beroes JM, Shekelle PG. Mental health conditions among patients seeking and undergoing bariatric surgery: a meta-analysis. *JAMA.* 2016; 315(2): 150–63.

51 Neovius M, Bruze G, Jacobson P, Sjöholm K, Johansson K, Granath F, et al. Risk of suicide and non-fatal self-harm after bariatric surgery: results from two matched cohort studies. *Lancet Diabetes Endocrinol.* 2018; 6(3): 197–207.

52 Lagerros YT, Brandt L, Hedberg J, Sundbom M, Bodén R. Suicide, self-harm, and depression after gastric bypass surgery: a nationwide cohort study. *Ann Surg.* 2017; 265(2): 235–43.

53 King WC, Chen J-Y, Mitchell JE, Kalarchian MA, Steffen KJ, Engel SG, et al. Prevalence of alcohol use disorders before and after bariatric surgery. *JAMA.* 2012; 307(23): 2516–25.

54 King WC, Chen J-Y, Courcoulas AP, Dakin GF, Engel SG, Flum DR, et al. Alcohol and other substance use after bariatric surgery: prospective evidence from a U.S. multicenter cohort study. *Surg Obes Relat Dis.* 2017; 13(8): 1392–402.

55 Steffen KJ, Engel SG, Wonderlich JA, Pollert GA, Sondag C. Alcohol and other addictive disorders following bariatric surgery: prevalence, risk factors and possible etiologies. *Eur Eat Disord Rev.* 2015; 23(6): 442–50.

56 Sogg S. Comment on: Alcohol and other substance use after bariatric surgery: prospective evidence from a us multicenter cohort study. *Surg Obes Relat Dis.* 2017; 13 (8): 1402–4.

Gender Incongruence
Key Considerations in Transitioning

Anne M. Doherty and Todd B. Nippoldt

Introduction

People who are transgender and gender non-conforming (TGNC) are those whose experienced gender is different from their assigned sex at birth, and they have specific healthcare needs.

As the number of people identifying as TGNC is increasing internationally, it is important that endocrinologists, psychiatrists and indeed all health professionals have a good understanding of issues related to the physical and mental healthcare of transgender people. People who identify as TGNC experience a disproportionate amount of violence, discrimination and stigma, and these factors contribute to poorer health outcomes. There is also a high rate of comorbidity in young people who are TGNC, including mood disorders, eating disorders, suicidal ideation and self-harm. Compounding these mental health problems are the effects of social exclusion (including from education and employment), which often places TGNC people at risk, especially during transitioning.

Diagnostic Classification

Different classification systems and descriptive terms have been used in recent years, and the terminology has evolved swiftly. *Gender identity disorder* is the diagnostic category used in both the Tenth Revision of the International Classification of Disease and Related Health Problems (ICD-10) and the *Diagnostic and Statistical Manual of Mental Disorders*, 4th edition (DSM-IV) (1, 2). In ICD-10, which remains the current classification system of the World Health Organization (WHO), this is included in the chapter on mental and behavioural disorders (chapter F). In DSM-5, the diagnosis is updated to *gender dysphoria*, which is described as a 'marked incongruence between one's experienced/expressed gender and assigned gender of at least 6 months' duration' and 'clinically significant distress or impairment in social, school, or other important areas of functioning' (3). Therefore, the presence of distress and dysfunction are central to its diagnosis in DSM-5, and its presence in DSM-5 keeps it defined as a mental disorder.

In the long anticipated ICD-11, due to be published in 2022, the gender identity disorder of ICD-10 categorised under psychiatric disorders will be replaced by *gender incongruence of adolescence and adulthood* and will be categorised under Conditions Related to Sexual Health (4). This change occurred in response not just to the evolving research and clinical-based knowledge available, but also on the basis of changes in law, policy and human rights standards, which had made the previous categorisation under mental and behavioural disorders increasingly controversial. In ICD-11, the primary focus will be on the incongruence between natal sex and experienced gender, rather than the distress or dysphoria associated with this under DSM-5: in ICD-11, dysphoria may be present but is not a requirement for a diagnosis of gender incongruence. As in the ICD-10, there is a restriction in the diagnosis of gender incongruence of adolescence and adulthood before the onset of puberty.

In ICD-11, the diagnostic requirements for gender incongruence of adolescence and adulthood will include the continuous presence for at least several months (a reduction from two years in ICD-10) of at least two of the following features:

(1) Strong dislike or discomfort with primary and/or secondary sexual characteristics due to their incongruity with the experienced gender.
(2) Strong desire to be rid of some or all of one's primary and/or secondary sexual characteristics (or, in adolescence, anticipated secondary sex characteristics).
(3) Strong desire to have the primary and/or secondary characteristics of the experienced gender.
(4) Strong desire to be treated (to live and be accepted as) a person of the experienced gender (4).

Epidemiology of Gender Incongruence

Gender incongruence, or gender dysphoria (previously known as gender identity disorder), is being identified with increasing frequency over the past two decades. The real prevalence rate is unknown, with few reliable epidemiological studies in the area, and the majority of figures quoted are extrapolated from numbers attending services.

The official prevalence rate published by the WHO in 1997 quoted a prevalence of 1 person in 60,000 (male = 1:30,000, female = 1:100,000). DSM-5, when it was published in 2013, quoted a prevalence rate three times greater of 1 person in 20,000 (male = 1:10,000, female = 1:30,000).

Collin et al. conducted a systematic review of the prevalence of gender incongruence and found that there was significant heterogeneity in the included studies, most of which were based on clinical populations. They subdivided the studies according to whether they (1) had undergone gender-affirming treatments such as hormone therapy and surgery, (2) had been given an ICD/DSM diagnosis or (3) self-identified as transgender (5). They found prevalence rates of completed surgery of 1/100,000 for trans women and 0.25/100,000 for trans men in the USA and of 35.2/100,000 for trans women and 12.0/100,000 for trans men in Singapore. On meta-analysis, this gave a prevalence estimate of 9.2/100,000 (12.5/100,000 among trans women and 5.1/10,000 among trans men). They found prevalence rates of documented ICD/DSM diagnoses of 0.69/100,000 for trans women and 0.74/100,000 for trans men in Iran, with the highest rates of trans women reported in the USA being 22.9/100,000 and 32.9/100,000 from the Veterans Health Association (differing methodology in the studies resulting in the different prevalence rates reported). On meta-analysis, this gave a prevalence estimate of 6.8/100,000 (5.8/100,000 among trans women and 2.5/10,000 among trans men). Collin et al. found six studies of wider populations who responded to surveys, with prevalence rates ranging from 100/100,000 to 7,300/100,000. However, it must be noted that some of these studies based this identification on very loose definitions: in one case, this was based on a positive answer to the question 'I wish I was the opposite sex'. On meta-analysis (excluding this one study), this gave a prevalence estimate of 355.1/100,000 (521.5/100,000 among trans women and 256.2/10,000 among trans men) (5).

Minority Stress and Its Consequences

Transgender people often experience gender dysphoria as a result of minority stress. Minority stress results from discrimination (experiences of prejudice), stigma (anticipation of negative social attitudes), internalised stigma (absorption of negative social attitudes) and microaggressions (6). In many societies, such as the USA, transgender people experience poverty, homelessness and unemployment at rates much higher than the general population. This translates into a marked increase in specific health risks, including depression, anxiety, self-harm, suicide, substance abuse, HIV and other sexually transmitted infections, emotional, physical and sexual abuse and delay or denial of healthcare (7). Microaggressions (everyday subtle, intentional or unintentional verbal or behavioural indignities that communicate bias towards historically marginalised groups) are widely experienced in the transgender population and contribute to the development of dysphoria. Misgendering (failure to use the affirmed name and pronouns) is a common microaggression transgender people experience. This can result in significant distress as it undermines the person's experience of gender. Basic civility, including referring to the person by their affirmed name and pronouns, can minimise the distress experienced. Where you are unsure of the pronouns used, it may be helpful to clarify by simply asking, 'What pronouns do you use?'

A UK-based survey published in 2019 reported that 40% of transgender people reported at least one negative experience with healthcare in the preceding year related to their gender identity (8). Where stigma is present in healthcare settings, it may be associated with barriers to transition, and even barriers to regular healthcare (9). Specific barriers to gender-affirming treatments, including hormone therapy, puberty suppression and surgery, have been reported by many patients. These can take the form of financial barriers, difficulties in accessing services and interpersonal barriers with healthcare professionals (10). It is essential that healthcare providers and the healthcare environment be consistently affirming of the TGNC patient to create a positive healthcare experience. This can include a welcoming waiting room, gender-inclusive restrooms, identification of the affirmed name and pronouns and their consistent use by all staff and in the medical record. The medical record and intake forms may need to be modified to ensure the collecting and documenting of this information correctly.

It is positive to note that attitudes towards transgender people are relatively positive in psychiatrists (11). Perhaps more tolerant attitudes towards minorities in society are contributing to this, and perhaps specific workplace-based training is a factor (12).

Many professional bodies have issued statements regarding conversion therapies, which aim to suppress the affirmed gender, recommending against their use. A systematic review examining conversion therapies and barriers to transition has demonstrated that there is no evidence of effectiveness (13).

Comorbid Mental Health Diagnoses

Transgender people are at higher risk of developing mental health difficulties. In the UK, patients attending a gender identity service who were not taking gender-affirming hormone treatment had four times the risk of depression compared with controls, and this was predicted by older age, poor interpersonal functioning, low self-esteem and reduced social support. Hormone treatments were associated in lower depression scores (14). A study from the National Inpatient Sample in the USA examined over 25,000 transgender inpatient encounters and over 250,000,000 cisgender inpatient encounters and reported a significantly greater proportion of mental disorders in the transgender group (77.0% compared with 37.8%). Transgender people had on odds ratio of 7.9 for all mental disorders, and odds ratios of 3.4 for anxiety, 1.6 for depression and 2.5 for psychosis (15). As many as 62% of transgender adults may have comorbid depressive illnesses (16, 17).

There is a growing prevalence (or perhaps awareness) of autistic spectrum disorders (ASDs) in patients referred for assessment among children, adolescents and adults. A recent systematic review found a higher prevalence rate of ASDs in transgender children and adolescents compared with the general population, but there is less conclusive evidence for this in adults (18).

There is evidence that psychometric tools for the assessment of personality factors are not validated in the transgender population (19). One study that conducted the Minnesota Multiphasic Personality Inventory before and after testosterone treatments in transgender men found significant improvements in problematic personality traits following treatment with testosterone (20).

Suicidal Ideations and Behaviours

Transgender people are at elevated risk of self-harm and suicide. Each individual will experience a different degree of dysphoria, related perhaps to their need for transition and the degree to which the dysphoria impacts on the various domains of functioning: social, occupational and family. Rates of suicidal ideations and behaviours in transgender populations are in the main derived from small studies of clinical populations, rather than from larger epidemiological studies, and there is thus some inherent bias to these rates.

There is significant variability reported in the incidence of self-harm among transgender people, which occurs at rates as high as 44%, significantly higher than the general population (21). Similarly, there is variability reported in the presence of symptoms of suicidal ideation among transgender people, ranging from 37% to 83% (22). Garcia-Vega et al. explored the methods of self-harm utilised in their cohort of 151 attendees at a specialist transgender clinic and found significant proportions of people attending reported a history of serious suicidal behaviours, including attempted hanging (6% of trans men), road traffic accident (2% of trans women) and jumping from a height (3% of trans women and 2% of trans men) (23).

The existing evidence suggests that there are elevated rates of completed suicide in transgender populations. In a systematic review, Marshall et al. found a completed suicide rate of 4.2%, but six of the studies reviewed only examined outcomes of people who had completed gender-affirming surgeries. They concluded that transgender people were at higher risk for suicidal ideations and behaviours than the general population and that trans men are at a higher risk than trans women (24). An 18.5-year cohort study of 1,331 transgender people in The Netherlands who had received hormonal treatment found a higher risk of completed suicide in trans women, with little difference in significance between trans men and the general population (25). A US-based study of over 2,600 patients found no significant difference in suicide rates between trans men and trans women, with the trans populations overall having a significantly higher risk of suicide (26). The largest cohort to date based in Amsterdam reported the outcomes of 5,107 trans men and 3,156 trans women and found 49 deaths by suicide (0.8% of trans women and 0.3% of trans men), which was three to four times the mortality rate of the Dutch population in the study period. The authors noted that suicide risk did not differ to a significant extent depending on the stage of transitioning (27).

The aetiology and underlying reasons why transgender people have higher rates of self-harm and suicide have been the subject of some research, and it is thought that comorbid mental disorders may contribute to some degree. Psychosocial factors, especially those relating to isolation and belongingness, may similarly contribute to the development of these thoughts and acts. In a study of suicidality in young transgender people, Austin et al. reported that interpersonal microaggressions and emotional neglect by their family of origin were associated with lifetime suicidality and that a sense of belonging at school, familial emotional neglect and self-stigma were associated with suicidality in the six-month period preceding the study (28).

Assessment

Multidisciplinary Team

Hembree et al. describe the requirements for a gender multidisciplinary team in the clinical practice guidelines published by the Endocrine Society, co-published with the American Association for Clinical Endocrinologists, the American Society of Andrology, the European Society for Paediatric Endocrinology, the European Society of Endocrinology, the Pediatric Endocrine Society and the World Professional Association for Transgender Health (29). These guidelines are clear about the multidisciplinary nature of transgender healthcare and in particular their endocrine treatment. They stipulate that an appropriately trained diagnosing clinician is required and that for adolescents a mental health provider is required, and one is recommended (but not required) for adults. The guidelines recommend that trained mental health professionals should diagnose gender dysphoria or gender incongruence in adults and that this diagnosing clinician must be competent to diagnose mental disorders, to diagnose gender dysphoria or gender incongruence and to differentiate from other conditions such as body dysmorphic disorder. The diagnosing clinician must be able to deliver or refer for any required treatments, to assess competence and any factors that might impact on understanding and to regularly attend appropriate professional meetings. The guidelines recommend that the mental health professionals diagnosing gender dysphoria or gender incongruence in children and adolescents must meet the above criteria, with specific training in the developmental psychology of children and adolescents, and they must also understand the criteria for the use of puberty-blocking and gender-affirming hormones (9).

It has been suggested that there are specific difficulties with mental health professionals being seen as gatekeepers of gender services. First, this conveys the idea that a person who is transgender has a primary mental disorder. Second, given that there is significant psychiatric comorbidity with gender incongruence, and given in particular the high rates of suicidal ideations and behaviours, it is essential that transgender people have good access to mental healthcare. If they feel that the mental healthcare provider is in a gatekeeping role, they may be reluctant to disclose difficulties out of fear that it may have implications for their progression towards gender-affirming treatments. Reassurance that the purpose of mental/behavioural health assessments is to optimise the outcomes of social, hormonal and surgical transition is essential.

The informed consent model rather than the diagnostic model of care has become increasingly topical in recent years. This model suggests that rather than focusing on a diagnosis of gender incongruence or gender dysphoria, the focus should be on the person's ability to give informed consent for gender-affirming treatments (30).

The assessment process must be robust in order to ensure safe and appropriate treatment for patients with gender incongruence or dysphoria. In addition to confirming the clarity and stability of the person's transgender identity, the assessment should explore the mental health and social factors that may pose a risk during transitioning and identify necessary care. The development of multidisciplinary team care within gender clinics has enhanced the quality of mental healthcare for patients with gender incongruence or dysphoria (31).

Social Gender Role Transitioning

For many transgender people, the first step in transitioning is the social gender role transition. This involves living as the identified gender, and it usually involved changing their name and pronouns. This will usually be associated with an adoption of the dress, hairstyles, make-up, etc., of the gender identity. Various techniques may be used to present the shape of the preferred gender, including the use of binders (used by trans men to present a flat chest), packers (used to present a male silhouette) or tucking (a technique used by trans women in order to make the genitals non-visible in tighter clothing).

This may be accompanied by legal changes to gender. In the UK, the Gender Recognition Act was passed in 2004, and it allows people to have a gender recognition certificate issued that updates the person's gender from that assigned at birth. Many other countries have similar legislation: in Ireland, the Gender Recognition Act was passed in 2015, while in the USA, Canada and Australia, the procedure varies considerably by state.

Endocrinology Management

The goal of feminising and masculinising hormone therapy is to relieve dysphoria by inducing physical and emotional changes that are consistent with the person's affirmed gender. The most recent World Professional Association for Transgender Health (WPATH) guidelines indicate that hormonal therapy can be started at a time at which any medical and mental health issues are under reasonable control. The medical evaluation includes a medical history, physical examination and often laboratory tests to identify and correct any conditions that may influence the choice of the specific medications, as well as dosages and routes of administration. The mental and behavioural health evaluation includes assessment of the control of any mental health diagnoses, as well as social issues that can influence the success of treatment, including financial and employment status, identifying a personal support system and any housing or travel issues. In addition, counselling and psychological support during hormonal transition is very beneficial for most patients. Such assessments and therapies are ideally accomplished by a separate mental health provider, and although they are desirable but not necessary according to WPATH standards, they remain as requirements in many individual gender clinics.

For male-to-female transitioning, feminising hormone therapy aims to diminish the production or block the effect of endogenous testosterone and provide feminisation with oestrogen. Testosterone-blocking drugs such as spironolactone are often used in conjunction with oestrogen, which suppresses testosterone levels in addition to providing feminisation. For female-to-male transitioning, masculinising hormone therapy is accomplished with testosterone that, in addition to providing masculinisation, suppresses ovarian function, resulting in lower levels of oestrogen and a cessation of menses. In some cases, suppression of the endogenous hormone is accomplished with a gonadotrophin-releasing hormone analogue, and this may allow for lower doses of the affirmed sex hormone. Other medications are often used in specific circumstances. Progesterone may improve breast development and emotional status in trans women and promote cessation of menses in trans men. 5-Alpha reductase inhibitors may be beneficial is reversing androgenic balding in trans women and prevent balding in trans men. With baseline medical investigation and ongoing monitoring, transitioning hormone therapy is relatively safe (see Table 11.1) (31). In some cases, transgender people may order hormones on the Internet – as these are unregulated and unlicensed and unaccompanied by monitoring, they carry significant risk.

Prior to commencing gender-affirming hormone therapy, transgender people should be counselled on the impact of hormone treatments on their fertility and offered fertility preservation options (31). Trans women may wish to avail of cryopreservation of sperm prior to initiating treatment. Trans men usually experience amenorrhoea following treatment with testosterone, which in many cases is reversible with cessation of testosterone treatment. Trans men may wish to avail of cryopreservation of oocytes, embryos or ovarian tissue, especially when gonadectomy is planned. In adolescents, pubertal suppression with gonadotrophin-releasing hormone analogues are often used. This allows time for gender exploration and affirmation while preventing the physical changes – many of which are irreversible – that occur with natal puberty. Discontinuation of gonadotrophin-releasing hormone analogues is reversible and, if masculinising or feminising hormone therapy is not started, the adolescent will proceed through natal puberty (32).

Further gender-affirming treatments include permanent hair removal (laser or electrolysis) and speech and language therapy to help achieve the vocal qualities of the identified gender.

Gender-Affirming Surgery

Gender-affirming surgery will be requested in a number of transgender people once established on hormone treatments. Not all transgender people will wish for surgery, and different people will wish to progress at different speeds.

Trans women may require genital surgeries that include penectomy, orchidectomy, vaginoplasty, cliteroplasty and labioplasty. In addition, while some people may have adequate breast tissue development with oestrogen, others may require breast augmentation. Some may require thyroid chondroplasty and facial feminising surgery.

Trans men will often be keen to have breast surgery (mastectomies and chest wall reconstruction) early in the process of transitioning. 'Bottom surgery' for trans men may include a number of the following: hysterectomy, salpingo-oophorectomy and vaginectomy and phalloplasty, metadoidioplasty, urethroplasty, scrotoplasty and testicular and erectile prostheses. The Endocrine Society guidelines suggest that genital gender-affirming surgery should proceed only after the endocrinologist (or other doctor prescribing hormones) and the mental health professional agree that it is medically necessary and would benefit the patient's well-being. The guidelines suggest that transgender patients should have completed at least one year of 'consistent and compliant' hormonal treatment (unless contraindicated or not desired) and should have achieved a 'satisfactory social role change' (29).

Table 11.1 A representative protocol for monitoring transgender hormone therapy.

	Baseline	Measure every 8–12 weeks while titrating to maintenance dose	Measure 6-monthly for first 3 years, then annually
Body mass index	X		X
Blood pressure	X		X
Full blood count	X		X
Urea and electrolytes	X		X
Liver function tests	X		X
Lipid profile	X		X
Fasting glucose and/ or HbA1c	X		X
Thyroid function tests	X		If abnormal
Prolactin	X		X
Trans women			
Testosterone	X	X	X
Oestradiol	X	X	X
Trans men			
Testosterone	X	X	X
Oestradiol	X		
Bone density measurement	Not unless specific indication		May be required for those who have had gonadectomy or where there are additional risk factors for osteoporosis

Managing Psychiatric Comorbidities

Any psychiatric comorbidities should be treated in accordance with the usual guidelines, but taking into account the increased risk of suicide in the transgender population and the presence of stressors based on marginalisation and stigma that may be specific to TGNC people.

The prevalence of mental illness and mental distress in this group greatly exceeds that of the general population, and the provision of expert, specialist mental healthcare can significantly reduce this burden and improve outcomes. These mental health problems are frequently improved by transitioning, and conversely delay in providing treatment can result in mental health problems, substance misuse and suicide. In some cases, however, ill-informed treatments can also lead to mental health deterioration, substance misuse and suicide. Therefore, psychiatric evaluation before commencing treatment and the availability of ongoing psychiatric input and psychological support during transitioning is essential to the safe delivery of a gender service.

In some clinics and jurisdictions, due to the established levels of psychiatric comorbidity, it is a requirement that a person with gender dysphoria receives two psychiatric opinions prior to commencing treatment in order to confirm the diagnosis and to identify any mental disorders that may require treatment.

Beyond Transition

Following transition, the guidelines recommend that people who have undergone gender-affirming treatments receive ongoing monitoring of hormone treatment and any post-surgical care that may be needed.

Transgender people must receive appropriate cancer screening based on the presence of the particular organ rather than on their gender. They should be enrolled in the necessary cancer screening programmes, and care is required that they are not removed following any changes in name or legal gender status. This should be based on the principle of targeting the organ (rather than the gender). In general, the recommended screening protocols in place for cis men and women apply to trans men and women. Trans men who have not had surgery to remove the cervix will require cervical cancer screening, and those who have not had mastectomy will require breast cancer screening. Trans women will require prostate cancer screening, and those on oestrogen therapy will require breast cancer screening. An older trans women should have screening for abdominal aortic aneurysm due to the risks she carries based on her natal sex. Transgender people may find having to undergo screening that is associated with natal sex rather than identified gender distressing, and every effort should be made to minimise the distress caused while ensuring appropriate screening occurs.

Conclusion

People who are transgender have specific healthcare needs. As the number of people identifying as TGNC is increasing internationally, it is important that endocrinologists, psychiatrists and indeed all health professionals have a good understanding of the issues related to the physical and mental healthcare of transgender people.

People who identify as TGNC experience a disproportionate amount of violence, discrimination and stigma, and these factors contribute to poorer health outcomes. There is also a high rate of mental health comorbidities in young people with gender incongruence or dysphoria. Compounding these mental health problems are the effects of social exclusion (including from education and employment), which often places TGNC people at risk, especially during transitioning. Transgender people should have access to expert guideline-based care that allows them to transition safely and to optimise their health and well-being.

References

1 WHO. *The ICD-10 Classification of Mental and Behavioural Disorders: Clinical Descriptions and Diagnostic*

Guidelines. World Health Organisation, 1992.

2 APA. *The Diagnostic and Statistical Manual of Mental Disorders*, 4th ed. (DSM-

IV). American Psychiatric Publishing, 1994.

3   APA. *The Diagnostic and Statistical Manual of Mental Disorders*, 5th ed. (DSM-5). American Psychiatric Publishing, 2013.

4   Reed GM, Drescher J, Krueger RB, Atalla E, Cochran SD, First MB, et al. Disorders related to sexuality and gender identity in the ICD-11: revising the ICD-10 classification based on current scientific evidence, best clinical practices, and human rights considerations. *World Psychiatry.* 2016; 15(3): 205–21.

5   Collin L, Reisner SL, Tangpricha V, Goodman M. Prevalence of transgender depends on the 'case' definition: a systematic review. *J Sex Med.* 2016; 13(4): 613–26.

6   Meyer IH. Minority stress and mental health in gay men. *J Health Soc Behav.* 1995; 36(1): 38–56.

7   James SE, Herman JL, Rankin S, Keisling M, Mottet L, Anafi MA. *The Report of the 2015 US Transgender Survey.* National Center for Transgender Equality, 2016.

8   Office GE. *National LGBT Survey Research Report.* UK Government Department for Education, 2018.

9   Safer JD, Coleman E, Feldman J, Garofalo R, Hembree W, Radix A, et al. Barriers to healthcare for transgender individuals. *Curr Opin Endocrinol Diabetes Obes.* 2016; 23(2): 168–71.

10   Puckett JA, Cleary P, Rossman K, Newcomb ME, Mustanski B. Barriers to gender-affirming care for transgender and gender nonconforming individuals. *Sex Res Social Policy.* 2018; 15(1): 48–59.

11   Ali N, Fleisher W, Erickson J. Psychiatrists' and psychiatry residents' attitudes toward transgender people. *Acad Psychiatry.* 2016; 40(2): 268–73.

12   Hunt R, Bates C, Walker S, Grierson J, Redsell S, Meads C. A systematic review of UK educational and training materials aimed at health and social care staff about providing appropriate services for LGBT+ people. *Int J Environ Res Public Health.* 2019; 16(24): 4976.

13   Wright T, Candy B, King M. Conversion therapies and access to transition-related healthcare in transgender people: a narrative systematic review. *BMJ Open.* 2018; 8(12): e022425.

14   Witcomb GL, Bouman WP, Claes L, Brewin N, Crawford JR, Arcelus J. Levels of depression in transgender people and its predictors: results of a large matched control study with transgender people accessing clinical services. *J Affect Disord.* 2018; 235: 308–15.

15   Hanna B, Desai R, Parekh T, Guirguis E, Kumar G, Sachdeva R. Psychiatric disorders in the U.S. transgender population. *Ann Epidemiol.* 2019; 39: 1–7.e1.

16   Clements-Nolle K, Marx R, Guzman R, Katz M. HIV prevalence, risk behaviors, health care use, and mental health status of transgender persons: implications for public health intervention. *Am J Public Health.* 2001; 91(6): 915–21.

17   Hoy-Ellis CP, Fredriksen-Goldsen KI. Depression among transgender older adults: general and minority stress. *Am J Community Psychol.* 2017; 59(3–4): 295–305.

18   Glidden D, Bouman WP, Jones BA, Arcelus J. Gender dysphoria and autism spectrum disorder: a systematic review of the literature. *Sex Med Rev.* 2016; 4(1): 3–14.

19   Lehmann K, Leavey G. Accuracy of psychometric tools in the assessment of personality in adolescents and adults requesting gender-affirming treatments: a systematic review. *Eur Psychiatry.* 2019; 62: 60–7.

20   Keo-Meier CL, Herman LI, Reisner SL, Pardo ST, Sharp C, Babcock JC. Testosterone treatment and MMPI-2 improvement in transgender men: a prospective controlled study. *J Consult Clin Psychol.* 2015; 83(1): 143–56.

21   Heylens G, Elaut E, Kreukels BP, Paap MC, Cerwenka S, Richter-Appelt H, et al. Psychiatric characteristics in transsexual individuals: multicentre study in four European countries. *Br J Psychiatry.* 2014; 204(2): 151–6.

22 McNeil J, Ellis SJ, Eccles FJR. Suicide in trans populations: a systematic review of prevalence and correlates. *Psychology of Sexual Orientation and Gender Diversity.* 2017; 4(3): 341–53.

23 Garcia-Vega E, Camero A, Fernandez M, Villaverde A. Suicidal ideation and suicide attempts in persons with gender dysphoria. *Psicothema.* 2018; 30(3): 283–8.

24 Marshall E, Claes L, Bouman WP, Witcomb GL, Arcelus J. Non-suicidal self-injury and suicidality in trans people: a systematic review of the literature. *Int Rev Psychiatry.* 2016; 28(1): 58–69.

25 Asscheman H, Giltay EJ, Megens JA, de Ronde WP, van Trotsenburg MA, Gooren LJ. A long-term follow-up study of mortality in transsexuals receiving treatment with cross-sex hormones. *Eur J Endocrinol.* 2011; 164(4): 635–42.

26 Reisner SL, White JM, Bradford JB, Mimiaga MJ. Transgender health disparities: comparing full cohort and nested matched-pair study designs in a community health center. *LGBT Health.* 2014; 1(3): 177–84.

27 Wiepjes CM, den Heijer M, Bremmer MA, Nota NM, de Blok CJM, Coumou BJG, et al. Trends in suicide death risk in transgender people: results from the Amsterdam Cohort of Gender Dysphoria study (1972–2017). *Acta Psychiatr Scand.* 2020; 141(6): 486–91.

28 Austin A, Craig SL, D'Souza S, McInroy LB. Suicidality among transgender youth: elucidating the role of interpersonal risk factors. *J Interpers Violence.* 2020; doi: 10.1177/0886260520915554.

29 Hembree WC, Cohen-Kettenis PT, Gooren L, Hannema SE, Meyer WJ, Murad MH, et al. Endocrine treatment of gender-dysphoric/gender-incongruent persons: an endocrine society clinical practice guideline. *J Clin Endocrinol Metab.* 2017; 102(11): 3869–903.

30 Cavanaugh T, Hopwood R, Lambert C. Informed consent in the medical care of transgender and gender-nonconforming patients. *AMA J Ethics.* 2016; 18(11): 1147–55.

31 WPATH. *Standards of Care for the Health of Transsexual, Transgender, and Gender-Nonconforming People, Version 7.* World Professional Association for Transgender Health, 2012.

32 Neblett MF, 2nd, Hipp HS. Fertility considerations in transgender persons. *Endocrinol Metab Clin North Am.* 2019; 48 (2): 391–402.

Chapter 2

Anti-androgens in Forensic Psychiatric Settings

Mary Davoren

Introduction to Endocrinology in Forensic Psychiatry

Endocrinologists may be asked to confer with psychiatrists from time to time concerning the treatment of people with paraphilias or sex offenders. Neither paraphilias nor sexual offences are necessarily medical or psychiatric matters. Any doctor may encounter such cases from time to time. Within psychiatry, forensic psychiatrists specialise in the assessment, treatment and liaison with courts for those accused of sexual offences or subsequently engaged in treatment for such matters. When medical specialists or physicians have concerns that patients attending their services may pose a risk of serious harm, it may be helpful to refer to a forensic psychiatrist.

Forensic psychiatrists often have a dual role: to treat mental disorder and to reduce violent recidivism (1). Forensic psychiatric services provide care and treatment to mentally disordered offenders in secure psychiatric hospitals, provide outpatient clinics to community patients who pose a high risk of harm to others and provide in-reach psychiatric clinics in prisons. Sexual offending and sexual violence exist on a spectrum, ranging from lower-grade offences, such as voyeurism and indecent exposure, to rape and sexual homicide. Forensic psychiatrists will mainly deal with higher-end offending, and biological treatment options are generally considered only for the most serious offenders.

Treatment of individuals with a history of sexual offending is challenging and typically combines psychiatric, psychological and criminal justice measures. Many of those reading the literature on the treatment of sexual offenders will find it strangely elusive. Psychological treatment approaches include both cognitive behavioural psychological treatment groups and psychodynamic interventions for individuals, both of which have a very limited research evidence base (2–4). The mainstay of treatment of sexual offenders in correctional settings consists of psychological group work, such as the sexual offender treatment programme (SOTP) in the UK (5). While some studies in relation to these interventions have been positive, on balance there is little research evidence to support these treatment groups. Recent studies have demonstrated no significant reduction in sexual reoffending or increased rates of reoffending among participants (6–8). Cochrane reviews have concluded that additional randomised controlled trials (RCTs) are needed in this area given the limited research evidence for these treatments at present (2). Therefore, in recent years, there has been an increased focus on the use of medication as an adjunct to psychosocial management in this group (9). The use of anti-androgen or testosterone-reducing medications should be carefully considered and is best jointly planned with a consultant forensic psychiatrist and endocrinologist. This chapter addresses the treatment of male sexual offenders. While females do perpetrate sexual offences (and this is under-reported), female sexual offenders are relatively rare and therefore the evidence base for treatment mainly concerns male offenders at this time.

Interest in the biological aspects of sexual offending is long-standing, as evidenced by Krafft-Ebbing's book *Psychopathia Sexualis* (1886) and the Danish castration 'experiments' of the early twentieth century (10, 11). Recidivism and reoffending were found even in the group that underwent castration in Denmark, and subsequently significant human rights questions were raised (11). The human rights aspects of castration and anti-androgen treatments are complex and cannot be ignored. Surgical castration of sexual offenders has not happened in Europe since the 1970s with the exception of Germany, where this persisted until 2012 with strict legal safeguards in place and on a voluntary basis only. Despite acknowledging the safeguards, this practice was criticised by the Committee for the Prevention of Torture (CPT) of the Council of Europe (12).

Epidemiology and Prevalence of Sexual Offending

Sexual violence is a significant public health issue, leading to high rates of morbidity and mortality worldwide each year (13). Victims suffer physical health problems, such as infectious diseases, injury, trauma, reproductive health issues, mental health issues such as mood disorders, and societal issues. Mortality associated with sexual violence includes suicide, murder and death from other causes such as AIDS (13). Sexual violence is a worldwide issue affecting adults and children, males and females. It also occurs in a wide variety of settings ranging from within marriages and families to conflict zones and refugee settings. Rates of sexual violence vary internationally, with lower rates typically reported from high-income countries (13). All types of sexual violence are known to be significantly under-reported to authorities, with sexual violence against male victims being very much under-reported (14, 15). The majority of sexual violence is not reported to the police. Of those incidents reported, a significant number do not progress to court and rates of conviction are low. Therefore, sexual violence conviction rates published by jurisdictions typically represent only a very small proportion of the true rate. This is the dark figure of sexual crime.[1] The true incidence of sexual violence is unknown.

Assessment of Sexual Offenders

History

The psychiatric assessment of sexual offenders should be undertaken by appropriately trained and experienced professionals, typically a consultant forensic psychiatrist or a highly experienced psychologist. The assessment must commence with a detailed history.

---

[1] The 'dark figure of crime' is a phrase from criminology that refers to the fact that most national crime statistics significantly underestimate the actual rate of crime in society. This is due to loss of crime figures on each step of the ladder: firstly, victims not reporting to the police; secondly, police not being in a position to have charges pressed; and finally, charges not resulting in convictions. The classic example is the research from the National Household Surveys, which ask members of the public to confidentially report violence they have committed. These surveys typically find crime rates that are multiples of the published government rates. This holds for most countries and also is especially true for sexual crimes, as these are known to be under-reported to a greater extent than other crimes.

This should include a past psychiatric history as well as a detailed biopsychosocial history assessing for traits of possible personality disorder. Very high rates of personality disorder are seen among individuals with a history of sexual offending, particularly those considered the highest-risk group (16, 17). However, this encompasses a wide variety of diagnostic categories, including dissocial, emotionally unstable, avoidant and schizoid personality disorders, among others (18, 19). A history of being a victim of trauma or sexual abuse as a child should also be noted. Psychopathy is associated with a high risk of recidivism in all offenders, and an assessment using the Psychopathy Checklist – Revised (PCL-R) may indicate callous, unemotional traits, which are relevant to sexual offending (18). Intellectual disabilities are developmental disorders and psychosexual development is complex. Therefore, it is not surprising that there are some individuals with neurodevelopmental disorders who engage in sexual violence towards others (20).

A lifetime substance misuse history should be carefully elicited. The patient is asked detailed questions about their use of substances such as alcohol, illicit drugs and novel psychoactive substances – from commencing the use of that substance to the daily pattern of use at the time of the offending behaviour, and after if this was a factor. A detailed psychosexual history should be taken, including early experiences, sexual preferences, past use of violence or coercion in sexual relationships, encounters with sex workers (and whether or not these included violence), sexual preferences for underage children and the genders and ages of the preferred sexual partners. Sexual attraction to inanimate objects and other paraphilias such as voyeurism and exhibitionism should also be explored. An enquiry about frequency of sexual activity, including masturbation, preoccupation, intrusiveness of arousing fantasies and the form and content of such fantasies, may be relevant when considering hormonal treatments.

A history of delinquency, acquisitive offending, fraud or physical violence without sexual components should also be documented. Most individuals who engage in sexual violence have a history of general violence and other rule-breaking behaviour. The pattern of violence and criminal behaviour should be documented over time, going through each successive charge and conviction to ascertain whether there is an escalating pattern to the offending.

When detailing the index offence, the assessor should note the age and gender of the victim or victims, preparations, precautions against discovery, concurrent use of substances and complexity of victim selection. High-density sexual offences (i.e. where a perpetrator commits a high number of crimes over a short time period), assaults on victims of multiple different types (e.g. different age groups and genders) and the use of weapons and death threats during the course of the assault are high-risk indicators. The degree of instrumentality of the violence is a key question. Other issues, such as the use of social media or Internet platforms to meet other offenders or share illegal material or to access potential victims, are important to document, as this information may be needed to manage and supervise the patient appropriately in the future in order to reduce the risk of reoffending. Misogynistic attitudes or attitudes that condone sexual offending should also be assessed.

The assessment of substance misuse histories and whether or not an individual was under the influence of alcohol or illicit drugs, including stimulant drugs, is very important. It is important to note that novel psychoactive substances, which are increasingly available, do not show up on most drug screens, and therefore a clear drug screen is unfortunately no longer an indication that intoxication was not a factor in any alleged offending behaviour. Voluntary intoxication does not mitigate intent before the law.

Police reports and criminal histories must be reviewed due to the possible unreliability of obtaining past forensic histories entirely from the interviewee. Collateral information in relation to behaviours, the use of violence and coercion within relationships and the use of substances is vital. A key aspect of the assessment of any individual with a history of sexual violence is a thorough assessment of the patients' willingness to engage in treatment and their wish to desist from offending behaviour. This can be difficult to assess prior to trial and sentencing. Patterns of denial in sex offenders are well documented and include those who admit their offence but 'rationalise' that it did not cause any harm to the victim, those who admit their offence but blame the victim, those who admit their offence but blame some temporary circumstances (e.g. their mental state or intoxication at the time) and lastly those who adamantly deny their offence (21). The first and final groups are the most unlikely to benefit from either psychological or medical treatment given the need to engage with either form of treatment on a longer-term basis in the community or in less supervised settings. A helpful approach at psychiatric interview includes a review of the book of evidence, including police and witness statements, in advance of the forensic psychiatric assessment, as this permits the assessor to make a determination regarding the accuracy or cognitive distortion of disclosures from the patient (21).

Instruments

The assessment of an individual with a history of sexual violence should be supported by the use of a structured risk assessment instrument. Violence risk assessment has evolved in forensic psychiatry from the use of unstructured clinical judgement, to the use of 'second-generation' actuarial instruments, to the use of third-generation structured professional judgement (SPJ) instruments (22). Unstructured clinical risk assessment is highly variable, with poor reliability, and it is clearly unsuitable for forensic settings where the risk to the public can be very high. Actuarial instruments were designed to improve on this by adding a score for a list of items statistically associated with the violent outcome. An example is the PCL-R (23). However, these instruments have the limitation of not including the clinical judgement of the assessing consultant. The SPJ approach is designed to incorporate the best of the actuarial approach with a list of evidence-based risk factors, combined with the clinician's judgement. Examples include Historical Clinical and Risk Management for Violence-20 (HCR-20), a very widely used violence risk assessment (24, 25). The aim of these risk assessment instruments is to focus on identifying factors associated with recidivism that are amenable to modification, as prediction of statistically rare outcomes is typically fraught with difficulties.

The most widely used assessment instruments for sexual offending include Static 99, the Risk for Sexual Violence Protocol (RSVP) and Sexual Violence Risk-20 (SVR-20) (26–28). All such instruments rely on the accuracy and completeness of the available information, the use of trained raters and methods being in place to ensure the ratings made conform to the definitions in the handbook of the SPJ instrument.

Capacity, Consent and Duress

A careful assessment of capacity, consent and potential duress issues must be undertaken. A formal assessment of capacity to consent to treatment with anti-androgens should be undertaken by or in conjunction with a consultant forensic psychiatrist prior to commencing any such treatment. Competent individuals have the right to consent to or refuse medical treatment, and it is the role of medical doctors to uphold this human right. Informed consent for treatment with anti-androgens requires the prescribing doctor to ensure the patient has been given adequate and detailed information about the possible benefits but also full disclosure about potential side effects, including the short- and long-term sequelae of accepting such treatment.

The role of duress is particularly challenging in this area. A patient may be of the view that a parole board or mental health tribunal may be more likely to sanction their release if they are in receipt of anti-androgen treatment. Thus, the use of an anti-androgen when the alternative is a lengthy prison sentence may blur the lines of voluntary consent. Medications such as anti-androgens have significant side effects. They may also be considered as interfering with bodily integrity. It is vital that the patient has a thorough understanding of the options they are weighing up. The assessment of consent to treatment should include a careful assessment of functional mental capacity to give or withhold consent to treatment. This requires an assessment of the patient's ability to understand information material to the decision, to reason about that information comparatively and consequentially and to reach a decision and communicate it while appreciating the importance of the information for themselves (29). A competent, capacitous patient may decide they would prefer release and freedom in the community when choosing the effects of an anti-androgen therapy compared to a prolonged incarceration.

Medical Treatment Options for Individuals with a History of Sexual Offending

There are a number of different biological treatment options for individuals with a history of sexual offending comprising in the main of two groups: medications to reduce libido and medications to reduce testosterone levels. Forensic psychiatrists often prefer medication given by long-acting injection because of its reliability. This may or may not be acceptable to the patient. Where these medications are prescribed orally or by other means, it is important to bear in mind that most studies of adherence to medication show large rates of non-compliance.

Selective Serotonin Reuptake Inhibitors and Antipsychotic Medications

Medications such as selective serotonin reuptake inhibitors (SSRIs) or antipsychotic medications reduce libido without directly reducing testosterone levels. SSRIs are associated with reduced sexual function, anorgasmia and difficulty with erection, and they were originally used to augment cognitive behavioural treatment programmes for individuals with a history of sexual offending (30). SSRIs inhibit 5-HT reuptake via antagonism of the serotonin transporter, which increases synaptic 5-HT. 5-HT reduces sexual function, and although the complete mechanism of this pathway remains unclear, it likely involves post-synaptic 5-HT_2. The use of an SSRI medication as a treatment option to reduce sexual drive in individuals with a history of serious sexual offending may be more acceptable to the patient, particularly if the patient has a comorbid history of a mood disorder such as depression or anxiety. SSRIs are generally well-tolerated medications. Most SSRI agents are associated with sexual dysfunction; however, there is evidence that the highest levels of sexual dysfunction are associated with paroxetine (31).

Antipsychotic Medications

Dopamine increases sexual dysfunction and therefore antipsychotic medications may reduce sexual drive (32). Antipsychotic medications can also increase prolactin, which has the effect of reducing sexual drive (33, 34). Antipsychotic medications have significant side effects. First-generation agents typically may give rise to extrapyramidal side effects and sedation. Second-generation agents have significant metabolic side effects such as weight gain leading to obesity, type 2 diabetes and other complications associated with raised body mass index, as described further in Chapter 3 (35, 36). Off-license prescriptions of antipsychotic medications for paraphilias or sexual offending should therefore be carefully considered. In individual patients where there are diagnoses of major psychotic illnesses and sexual offending, antipsychotic agents may have a useful therapeutic overlap, and it is advised that they should only be considered if the patient has a comorbid psychotic illness requiring antipsychotic therapy (37).

Oestrogens and Medroxyprogesterone

The use of oestrogens and medroxyprogesterone is likely to have a feminising effect, which will influence the extent to which these treatments are effective or acceptable for individual patients. Physical effects may include changes in body habitus that may be ego-syntonic or ego-dystonic. Psychological effects may or may not involve suppressing testosterone-driven libido and fantasy.

Medical treatment for sexual offenders with oestrogens may have significant side effects, including an increased risk of cardiovascular disease and breast cancer, although they are not associated with bone loss or osteoporosis (38). Balancing the potential benefits and significant side effects, they are not recommended for the treatment of men with sexual offending due to the weak evidence base.

Cyproterone Acetate and Gonadotrophin-Releasing Hormone Analogues

The aim of reducing blood testosterone levels in this population is to reduce libido and to reduce the frequency and intrusiveness of deviant sexual fantasies. It is worth bearing in mind that anabolic steroids and medicinal testosterone replacement can be associated with misuse, leading to irritability, aggression and hypersexuality. Both cyproterone acetate and gonadotrophin-releasing hormone (GnRH) analogues can cause temporary testosterone flares at the commencement of treatment, and it is therefore important to monitor patients for such symptoms in the early days of treatment.

Cyproterone acetate is a true anti-androgen. In most jurisdictions, it is licensed for the treatment of prostatic carcinoma. When used for the treatment of sexual offending, it is an off-license treatment and therefore due caution should be taken prior to commencing this treatment. Although available in long-acting injection and tablet forms, this medication should always be commenced orally. This is to allow titration against blood testosterone, but it is also due to a well-described initial surge of testosterone on commencement of treatment. Because this is a true testosterone antagonist, cyproterone acetate is widely believed to be effective in suppressing libido and fantasy. It is anecdotally said to be particularly effective at alleviating deviant fantasies. It is sometimes prescribed for a limited period of time to interrupt a cycle of deviant fantasy and masturbation in order to facilitate the commencement of psychological therapy addressing these issues. However, in most cases, transition from oral medication to long-acting injections should be considered. Regular monitoring of blood testosterone is necessary because of the common development of tolerance over time. It is particularly important to warn patients about the serious side effects of this medication, including potential liver damage. It is good practice always to give patients a copy of the product license insert to take away and read and to allow for a cooling-off period before the next clinic visit where this treatment is due to commence and before finalising consent.

GnRH is produced in the neurons of the hypothalamus and is the initial link in the hypothalamic–pituitary–gonadal axis, stimulating the production of follicle-stimulating hormone (FSH) and luteinising hormone (LH). GnRH analogue administration results in an initial flush of testosterone production; however, ongoing steady levels of GnRH analogues result in pituitary receptors becoming insensitive to LH and a downregulation of the pituitary–gonadal axis (39). Agents include leuprorelin, triptorelin, histrelin and goserelin. Clinicians administering this medication should note that there is an initial rise in testosterone over the first days, followed by a steady reduction, and testosterone levels should be at castration level (<20–50 ng/dL) within approximately one month (40). These medications are associated with significant side effects, including gynaecomastia, reduction in testicular volume and, importantly, reduction in bone density and potential effects on fertility (9). However, studies among patients with a history of sexual offending have demonstrated reductions in sexual fantasies and sexual behaviours, and the effects of the drugs are reversible on discontinuation (9). Due to the significance of the side-effect profile, it is recommended that GnRH analogues are considered only for the highest-risk offenders; however, good results were found in a maximum security hospital group (40, 41). While taking treatment with GnRH analogues, regular monitoring of testosterone levels and two-yearly assessment of bone density with dual-energy X-ray absorptiometry (DEXA) scans are recommended.

Ethical and Legal Issues for the Use of Testosterone-Reducing Medications

All medications to reduce sexual drive or testosterone levels in sexual offenders are off-license prescriptions. It is therefore very important that these are prescribed by consultants with the relevant level of experience and expertise in the area. It is important to clarify that the prescriber is covered by state or private indemnity in relation to these treatments. However, psychological interventions and interventions based on talking therapy for sexual offenders are also not without side effects. They are expensive to run in terms of therapist time and, given the results of systematic studies of their efficacy, they can falsely reassure probation services, community forensic teams and parole panels that a patient is ready for release to the community. The human rights implications of detaining individuals in secure settings such as prisons for non-completion of a treatment group with such a limited evidence base may, at times, be questionable. In relation to the rather limited research evidence base, this is likely due to the significant difficulties of running RCTs in secure settings, such as secure forensic hospitals or prisons. A second reason for the limited evidence base is the difficulty with developing accurate outcome measures for such RCTs. The most important outcome would clearly be recidivism in the area of sexual violence; however, given the under-reporting of sexual violence and the fact that these incidents are statistically rare occurrences, it would be difficult for an RCT to accurately assess the true rate of reoffending.

Conclusion

The assessment and treatment of paraphilias and sex offenders is highly complex. The limited evidence base for treatment extends to both psychological and talking therapy interventions, as well as biological and medication-based interventions. Biological interventions and medical management of sexual offending is a particularly challenging area. Evidence is only at the emerging stage in this area, and Cochrane reviews have advised that further research is required. Nonetheless, given the serious outcomes of potential risks to the patient, such as prolonged stays in secure settings, and to the public in the event of recidivism, medication can be considered in the highest-risk groups. Such treatment regimens require careful assessment, consideration and ongoing management. Consent and motivation for treatment in the individual patient are key to the success or failure of an intervention with such anti-libidinal medications, as the patient will need to voluntarily comply with this treatment in the community in the medium or long term. Patients who find their intrusive sexual thoughts ego-dystonic are probably the most suitable candidates for consideration for such treatment. It is therefore appropriate that such treatments are offered to the highest-risk offenders only.

References

1 Williams HK, Senanayke M, Ross CC, Bates R, Davoren M. Security needs among patients referred for high secure care in Broadmoor Hospital England. *BJPsych Open.* 2020; 6(4): e55.

2 Dennis JA, Khan O, Ferriter M, Huband N, Powney MJ, Duggan C. Psychological interventions for adults who have sexually offended or are at risk of offending. *Cochrane Database Syst Rev.* 2012; (12): CD007507.

3 Jones E, Chaplin E. A systematic review of the effectiveness of psychological approaches in the treatment of sex offenders with intellectual disabilities. *J Appl Res Intellect Disabil.* 2017; 33(1): 79–100.

4 Hanson RK. Review: evidence does not support a reduction in sexual reoffending with psychological interventions, but further high-quality trials are needed. *Evidence Based Ment Health.* 2013; 16(3): 68.

5 Marques JK, Day DM, Nelson C, West MA. Effects of cognitive behavioral treatment on sex offender recidivism: preliminary results of a longitudinal study. *Crim Justice Behav.* 1994; 21(1): 28–54.

6 Brown P, Ross C. Academic oversight in policy research: questions arising from the Sex Offender Treatment Programme study. *Lancet Psychiatry.* 2020; 7(3): 224–6.

7 Grady MD, Edwards D, Pettus-Davis C, Edwards D, Jr. A longitudinal outcome evaluation of a prison-based sex offender treatment program. *Sex Abuse.* 2017; 29(3): 239–66.

8 Mews A, Di Bella L, Purver M. *Impact Evaluation of the Prison-based Core Sex Offender Treatment Programme.* Ministry of Justice, 2017.

9 Alexandra L, Don G, Callum CR, Mrigendra D. Gonadotrophin-releasing hormone agonist treatment for sexual offenders: a systematic review. *J Psychopharmacol.* 2017; 31(10): 1281–93.

10 Krafft-Ebing RV. *Psychopathia Sexualis, with Especial Reference to Antipathetic Sexual Instinct: A Medico-forensic Study.* W. T. Keener and Co., 1900.

11 Le Louis M. Danish experiences regarding the castration of sexual offenders. *Journal of Criminal Law, Criminology, and Police Science.* 1956; 47(3): 294–310.

12 European Committee for the Prevention of Torture and Inhuman or Degrading Treatment or Punishment. *Report to the*

German Government on the Visit to Germany Carried Out by the European Committee for the Prevention of Torture and Inhuman or Degrading Treatment or Punishment. Council of Europe, 2012.

13 Krug EG, Mercy JA, Dahlberg LL, Zwi AB. The world report on violence and health. *Lancet.* 2002; 360(9339): 1083–8.

14 Brooks O, Burman M. Reporting rape: victim perspectives on advocacy support in the criminal justice process. *Criminol Crim Justice.* 2017; 17(2): 209–25.

15 Stemple L, Meyer IH. The sexual victimization of men in America: new data challenge old assumptions. *Am J Public Health.* 2014; 104(6): e19–26.

16 Fazel S, Sjöstedt G, Långström N, Grann M. Severe mental illness and risk of sexual offending in men: a case–control study based on Swedish national registers. *J Clin Psychiatry.* 2007; 68(4): 588–96.

17 Coid J, Yang M, Ullrich S, Zhang T, Roberts A, Roberts C, et al. *Predicting and Understanding Risk of Re-offending: The Prisoner Cohort Study. Research Summary.* Ministry of Justice, 2007.

18 Cardona N, Berman AK, Sims-Knight JE, Knight RA. Covariates of the severity of aggression in sexual crimes: psychopathy and borderline characteristics. *Sex Abuse.* 2020; 32(2): 154–78.

19 Dudeck M, Spitzer C, Stopsack M, Freyberger H, Barnow S. Forensic inpatient male sexual offenders: the impact of personality disorder and childhood sexual abuse. *J Forensic Psychiatry Psychol.* 2007; 18(4): 494–506.

20 Lindsay WR, Smith AHW, Law J, Quinn K, Anderson A, Smith A, et al. A treatment service for sex offenders and abusers with intellectual disability: characteristics of referrals and evaluation. *J Appl Res Intellect Disabil.* 2002; 15(2): 166–74.

21 Kennedy H, Grubin D. Patterns of denial in sex offenders. *Psychol Med.* 1992; 22(1): 191–6.

22 Hart SD, Logan C. Formulation of violence risk using evidence-based assessments: the structured professional judgment approach. In: *Forensic Case Formulation* (eds. P Sturmey, M McMurran). Wiley, 2011, pp. 83–106.

23 Hare RD. *The Psychopathy Checklist – Revised.* Pearson Clinical, 2003.

24 Webster CD. *HCR-20: Assessing Risk for Violence*, 2nd ed. Mental Health, Law, and Policy Institute, Simon Fraser University, in cooperation with the British Columbia Forensic Psychiatric Services Commission, 1997.

25 Douglas KS, Webster CD, Hart SD, Belfrage H. *HCR-20v3: Assessing Risk for Violence: User Guide*, 3rd ed. Mental Health, Law, and Policy Institute, Simon Fraser University, 2013.

26 Hanson RK, Thornton D. *Static 99: Improving Actuarial Risk Assessments for Sex Offenders.* Solicitor General Canada Ottawa, 1999.

27 Hart SD, Boer DP. Structured professional judgment guidelines for sexual violence risk assessment. In: *Handbook of Violence Risk Assessment* (eds. RK Otto, KS Douglas). Routledge, 2010, pp. 269–94.

28 Sutherland AA, Johnstone L, Davidson KM, Hart SD, Cooke DJ, Kropp PR, et al. Sexual violence risk assessment: an investigation of the interrater reliability of professional judgments made using the Risk for Sexual Violence Protocol. *Int J Forensic Ment Health.* 2012; 11(2): 119–33.

29 Appelbaum PS, Grisso T. The MacArthur Treatment Competence Study. I: Mental illness and competence to consent to treatment. *Law Hum Behav.* 1995; 19(2): 105–26.

30 Grubin D. Sexual offending and treatment of sex offenders. *Psychiatry.* 2004; 3(11): 17–21.

31 Jing E, Straw-Wilson K. Sexual dysfunction in selective serotonin reuptake inhibitors (SSRIs) and potential solutions: a narrative literature review. *Ment Health Clin.* 2016; 6 (4): 191–6.

32 Serretti A, Chiesa A. A meta-analysis of sexual dysfunction in psychiatric patients

taking antipsychotics. *Int Clin Psychopharmacol.* 2011; 26(3): 130–40.

33 Bancroft J. The endocrinology of sexual arousal. *J Endocrinol.* 2005; 186(3): 411–27.

34 Knegtering H, Van Der Moolen A, Castelein S, Kluiter H, Van Den Bosch R. What are the effects of antipsychotics on sexual dysfunctions and endocrine functioning? *Psychoneuroendocrinology.* 2003; 28: 109–23.

35 Miller DD, Caroff SN, Davis SM, Rosenheck RA, McEvoy JP, Saltz BL, et al. Extrapyramidal side-effects of antipsychotics in a randomised trial. *Br J Psychiatry.* 2008; 193(4): 279-88.

36 Rummel-Kluge C, Komossa K, Schwarz S, Hunger H, Schmid F, Lobos CA, et al. Head-to-head comparisons of metabolic side effects of second generation antipsychotics in the treatment of schizophrenia: a systematic review and meta-analysis. *Schizophr Res.* 2010; 123(2–3): 225–33.

37 Thibaut F, Barra FDL, Gordon H, Cosyns P, Bradford JMW. The World Federation of Societies of Biological Psychiatry (WFSBP) guidelines for the biological treatment of paraphilias. *World J Biol Psychiatry.* 2010; 11(4): 604–55.

38 Smith MR. Treatment-related osteoporosis in men with prostate cancer. *Clin Cancer Res.* 2006; 12(20 Pt 2): 6315s–9s.

39 Kumar P, Sharma A. Gonadotropin-releasing hormone analogs: understanding advantages and limitations. *J Hum Reprod Sci.* 2014; 7(3): 170–4.

40 Turner D, Briken P. Treatment of paraphilic disorders in sexual offenders or men with a risk of sexual offending with luteinizing hormone-releasing hormone agonists: an updated systematic review. *J Sex Med.* 2018; 15(1): 77–93.

41 Ho DK, Kottalgi G, Ross CC, Romero-Ulceray J, Das M. Treatment with triptorelin in mentally disordered sex offenders: experience from a maximum-security hospital. *J Clin Psychopharmacol.* 2012; 32(5): 739–40.

Chapter 3

Service- and Setting-Related Challenges

Residential Care and Inpatient Settings

13

Anne M. Doherty and Seán F. Dinneen

Introduction

Given the high rates of diabetes comorbid with many mental health conditions, it is no surprise that diabetes has a high prevalence in mental health facilities and settings. People with severe mental illness (SMI) die on average 17 years younger than the general population. When this 'mortality gap' is considered, along with the fact that cardiovascular diseases (including diabetes as a cardiovascular risk factor) contribute greatly to this mortality gap, the importance of acting to reduce incident diabetes and especially poorly controlled diabetes in these settings is clear. Specific measures may be required to ensure that patients in these settings receive the usual standard of diabetes care. There may be factors such as acuity of mental illness, lack of insight into both mental and physical health problems and practical difficulties in attending appointments that may mitigate against optimal diabetes management.

In this chapter, we will consider challenges that are specific to various settings, and we will also consider measures that may help to overcome or at least ameliorate these barriers to optimal care.

Acute Inpatient Mental Health Units

People admitted to most adult inpatient mental health units will have many of the conditions discussed in earlier chapters. Some will have acute depressive illnesses, some will have been admitted following serious suicide attempts and the vast majority will have been admitted with the first onset or a relapse of SMI. Many in the latter category will have a diagnosis of psychotic disorder, and many will be prescribed atypical antipsychotic agents. The nature of mental disorder, especially acute mental illness, means that patients will often have profound disturbances in their mood, in their thinking and in their perception, which may make it very difficult to maintain or to optimise their diabetes control. For example, patients may be paranoid about staff and may not wish to comply with any form of blood monitoring or other treatments. In these cases, stabilising their mental status is the first step towards optimising adherence to physical health treatments.

A meta-analysis of the prevalence of diabetes in inpatient mental health settings found an overall prevalence of 10%, with 90% of these having type 2 diabetes and the remaining 10% having type 1 diabetes (1). If patients are in hospital for a long period of time, they may miss screening opportunities (e.g. annual checks, including retinal screening). As a result, it is very important that the staff in adult mental health facilities are aware of these components of diabetes care and are able to ensure that patients remain up to date with all screening while in an inpatient setting (2).

Guidelines developed by the Joint British Diabetes Societies (JBDS) and the Royal College of Psychiatrists (RCPsych) suggest that best practice would involve the development of diabetes registers to include all patients in the mental health service (2). While arrangements would differ depending on the clinical setting, such an initiative may facilitate effective liaison with other facilities, such as retinal screening. The guidelines suggest that it may be helpful to have a named member of staff responsible for ensuring that as many of the required care processes as set out in the National Institute for Health and Care Excellence (NICE) guidelines can take place as indicated (3, 4). There may be benefits to having good local connections and relationships between mental health teams and the diabetes service. The JBDS/RCPsych guidelines suggest that diabetes management should be included in continuing professional development for members of mental health teams across disciplines (2). Inpatient units may consider dietetics' informed meal plans, that the design of menus will ensure the food served meets the needs of people with diabetes (as well as people with prediabetes and metabolic syndrome) and that portion sizes are suitable.

Each unit may need to consider how they will implement regular glucose monitoring for people with diabetes. Finally, it is important to consider the effects of individual antipsychotics on both risk of diabetes and glycaemic control in established diabetes and to consider the risks and benefits of prescribing on a case-by-case basis (5).

Residential/Long-Stay Mental Healthcare Facilities

Patients who live in long-term mental health facilities usually have SMI. Mental health staff in long-stay settings, including hostels (usually houses where three to four people with SMI live, with differing levels of staff involvement depending on the needs of the residents), have a similar role to those in inpatient settings, as they will often have daily contact with patients. Staff are in a position to remind patients to take their medications or supervise if needed. They may be able to help patients to incorporate activity and health checks into their routine. They are in a powerful position to advocate for their patients and to ensure that they have access to all needed physical healthcare.

Mental health facilities may wish to consider implementing screening programmes to allow them to identify undiagnosed diabetes. This will inform the management of diabetes in people who have been diagnosed. How such a screening programme is implemented and supported by the mental health service will depend on the needs of the local population. This may include screening everybody on admission using HbA1c fasting blood glucose or at intake to the service, and at regular intervals thereafter: the American Diabetes Association (ADA) suggests this testing should occur annually for people treated with antipsychotic medications (6). This happens automatically in patients who are prescribed clozapine: they regularly undergo testing of physical health parameters, including glucose (7). However, despite the ADA guidelines, this does not happen routinely other than with the mandated clozapine checks (8).

Structured diabetes education programmes are a key component of diabetes management. Diabetes Education and Self-Management for Ongoing and Newly Diagnosed (DESMOND) is one such programme for people with newly diagnosed type 2 diabetes, which is delivered widely as a basic component of care in the UK and Ireland. A randomised controlled trial of a specially adapted educational programme for people with psychosis did not demonstrate effectiveness (9). In delivering educational courses such as DESMOND, Dose Adjustment for Normal Eating (DAFNE; for type 1 diabetes) or similar programmes for people with SMI, it is worth taking into consideration the impact of illness (on concentration, interest, energy, etc.) and the patients' levels of literacy. It may be useful to include formal and informal carers, who will be able to later reinforce the education, and to consider a heavy focus on signposting healthy lifestyle tips and resources (2).

Secure Mental Health Settings

Diabetes is common in secure settings, with prevalence rates in adult forensic inpatient units of 14% being reported (10). The forensic mental health population is more likely to have severe forms of mental illness that may be treatment resistant. Many patients will be prescribed multiple antipsychotics, perhaps at very high doses. In addition, many patients in these settings will have spent several years institutionalised in secure hospitals or residential care. There is little research into the quality of diabetes care in these settings (2). It is important for any diabetes teams involved in the care of patients in these setting to appreciate the limitations of the forensic environment. For example, monitoring of blood glucose can only be undertaken by healthcare professionals, as patients cannot be given lancets for glucose testing. In addition, there may be restricted opportunities for exercise due to required levels of therapeutic security, with potentially restricted meal choices and difficulties in scheduling diabetes education.

Learning Disability or Intellectual Disability Units

There are no studies of the prevalence of diabetes in learning disability units; however, we know that people with learning disabilities are at a greater disadvantage when it comes to receiving healthcare and are more likely to die prematurely compared to the general population. There is a higher prevalence of type 2 diabetes and poorer outcomes in this population, partly due to institutionalisation, lack of exercise and a lack of targeted health promotion, and some groups may have a genetic predisposition (such as people with Down syndrome). Furthermore, limitations in social capabilities and literacy may hamper the generalisability of standard structured education to this population, creating a further disadvantage. There is emerging evidence that education programmes need to be modified to suit the needs of people with learning disabilities.

Long-Term Care

In Chapter 8, we discussed the specific difficulties relating to cognitive impairment and diabetes. Patients who live in residential or nursing care homes, such as those in inpatient settings, are in daily contact with nursing staff. Nursing home staff will be responsible for ensuring that patients attend their appointments with both mental health and physical health providers and will also be in a position to ensure that they attend for screening. In some instances, staff may be required to supervise and/or administer insulin and other long-acting injectable medications. They may need to supervise and administer oral medications and they may directly check blood glucose levels. They need to be confident in managing episodes of hypoglycaemia but also episodes of hyperglycaemia, including sick-day rules when patients have concomitant infections. Despite these expectations on nursing home staff, the reality is that quite often deficits exist in the training of nursing home staff and in their confidence and competence with delivering diabetes care (11). As a result, specialist diabetes nursing teams in hospitals are often contacted about day-to-day management, adding to the burden on the specialist function.

Antipsychotic Medications

Antipsychotic stewardship is a very important consideration. When somebody has an SMI, addressing this is the key priority for the optimisation of their overall health and functioning. However, if there is a way of treating this that is minimally diabetogenic, then this should be considered. The choice of medication needs to carefully weigh the risks and benefits of the treatment and its sequelae. Some of the most effective antipsychotic medications are those that carry the greatest risk of metabolic side effects, such as clozapine and olanzapine (12). When patients are being commenced on atypical antipsychotic medications they should be informed of the risk of diabetes and the risk of associated cardiovascular sequelae (13).

In instances where diabetogenic antipsychotics cannot be avoided, such as in the treatment of resistant psychosis where clozapine is indicated, it may be worth considering adjunctive medications that may reduce the risk of developing metabolic syndrome. A meta-analysis of the addition of metformin for antipsychotic-induced weight gain reported that this is an effective strategy for reducing the weight gain associated with antipsychotic treatment (14). Topiramate may also have some promise, although is likely to be less effective than metformin (15). A more recent meta-analysis of the effect of metformin on antipsychotic-induced dyslipidaemia reported significant improvements in low-density lipoprotein cholesterol, total cholesterol, triglycerides and high-density lipoprotein cholesterol and led to significant improvements in weight, body mass index, HbA1c, fasting insulin and insulin resistance (16). Antipsychotic medications are examined in more detail in Chapter 3.

Glucagon-like peptide-1 (GLP-1) receptor agonists may also have promise in weight reduction for people taking antipsychotic medications, as suggested by the randomised controlled trial of Svensson et al. (17). In addition to their weight-lowering effects, there may be improvements in glucose tolerance, low-density lipoprotein cholesterol, waist circumference and systolic blood pressure, as reported in the randomised controlled trial of Larsen et al. (18). There is emerging evidence that GLP-1 receptor agonists may also have antidepressant properties (19), but this has not been consistently reported: Gamble et al. reported no change in depressive symptoms and suicidal behaviours in a registry-based study (20). There are animal models that suggest that GLP-1 receptor agonists may have antipsychotic effects, although it remains to be seen whether this effect will be observed in human trials (21).

Organisational and Service Considerations

One of the barriers to good diabetes care for people with SMI is the configuration of services: the provision of mental and physical healthcare tends to occur in silos, with few organisational links, except where clinicians have intentionally created them. Better communication will help to optimise diabetes care and should be considered a priority where possible. This is particularly important when it comes to the management of diabetic emergencies such as diabetic ketoacidosis (DKA) and hyperglycaemic hyperosmolar state.

The JBDS/RCPsych guidelines suggest using a measure similar to the UK National Diabetes Inpatient Audit (NaDIA; which provides a snapshot of diabetes management among medical inpatients) in psychiatric inpatient settings to demonstrate the need for collaborative care, and indeed for basic diabetes care, in this population (22).

Key workers, care coordinators or primary mental health nurses have very close relationships in the community with patients with SMI. Accordingly, they may be key people to involve in training regarding the management of diabetes, as they will be well situated to help prompt and support the patient in the management of their diabetes.

Training Staff on Encouraging Adherence

Mental health staff, both in the community but more especially in inpatient settings, are well situated to encourage and support patients with the management of their physical health conditions. In the community, mental health staff will have regular contact with patients, perhaps weekly or even more frequently, and inpatient units will have continual staff presence, so this is a good opportunity to engage the patient in physical healthcare, and this might be regarded as a window of opportunity to address needs that might not otherwise be addressed. It is essential that systems are in place to facilitate the optimisation of this opportunity for patients in order to allow them not only to improve their mental health (care), but to also improve their physical health (care). Too often during the period of admission to mental health facilities is a patient's physical health negatively impacted: they may take up smoking, they may become more sedentary and they may be lethargic due either to altered mental state or prescribed medications, and as a result they find it more difficult to engage in physical activity. It is essential that all relevant members of the multidisciplinary teams are aware of their potential impact: psychiatrists have a part to play as the doctors on the team who have a responsibility towards mental and physical healthcare; mental health nurses are the professionals who see the patients most frequently and are in the best position to remind patients of diabetes management, activity, etc., during the day; occupational therapists may be able help optimise the patients' activity to incorporate physical activity and also self-care into their daily lives; psychologists may wish to include an adherence focus into any psychological therapies they are delivering, as there is evidence for the use of adherence-focused cognitive behavioural therapy; and finally, in settings where there is a pharmacist as part of the multidisciplinary team, their expertise in advising on medications and combinations of medications for patients with comorbid diabetes (or who are at risk of developing diabetes) will be valuable. Practically, it may be best to consider all patients in inpatient psychiatric settings to be at high risk of diabetes. Issues of adherence are discussed in more detail in Chapter 7.

Administering Insulin in the Inpatient Setting

One specific aspect of inpatient care that can be challenging is the administration of insulin, a drug that, if not administered correctly, can lead to serious morbidity and even mortality. In settings where patients may have limited ability to self-administer insulin, it may be of benefit to have staff trained to administer it. In the Southern Health NHS Foundation Trust in the UK, an initiative to train care staff to administer inulin to patients with learning disabilities successfully trained over 100 non-medical, non-nursing staff (23). This study did not report any impact on glycaemic control. The Making Insulin Treatment Safer (MITS) project is a prize-winning healthcare professional education programme geared towards Foundation-level doctors that aims to help prescribers analyse significant events related to insulin prescribing and get 'debriefed' on these by a trained debriefer. Developed by a group at Queen's University Belfast, the approach is based on empowerment theory to help junior doctors commit to safe future behaviour. This approach could easily be adapted to other healthcare settings (24).

Dieticians and Dietary Considerations

Access to dietetic advice and input may vary across the settings described above. In some settings, patients may not be able to attend the usual clinical settings for dietician review. In residential settings, there may be limited options for patients to select their food – in these cases, dietician-informed meal plans and advice regarding portion sizes will be especially important. Mental health settings may consider having their own in-house dietician who can tailor dietetic advice to the population (25). There may be particular benefit in dietetic-delivered tailored educational interventions; although little has been published in this area, an audit from Australia found significant benefits in terms of weight reduction in people with diabetes and SMI (26). When dietetic input is delivered as part of a broader programme it can achieve significant results (27).

Children and Adolescents

At any age receiving a diagnosis of diabetes is a life-changing event and, by definition, a stressor, and as such it may have an impact on the mental well-being of any person who has been diagnosed with diabetes. This is especially the case in children and young adults, where it can have a lasting impact on the child and their parents (28). Although few children with type 1 diabetes will meet the criteria for formal diagnosis of a mental disorder, many will experience various degrees of psychological distress. Diabetes distress can be conceptualised as the negative emotional burden of living with diabetes (29), and it can often be elevated in young people (30). This may be disabling and may have a detrimental effect on the self-management of their diabetes. As mentioned in Chapter 4, young women with diabetes are six times more likely to die than age-matched peers, and rates of suicide are also increased (31). Psychological and social factors are closely associated with premature death in type 1 diabetes. Many diabetes centres will have specific psychologists for children and adolescents both in the paediatric clinics and also through the ages where they transition to adult services. Transition from paediatric services to adult services is a difficult time for young people attending services for mental as well as physical healthcare, and managing this transition better has been a focus of many services and in research (32). In the Diabetes Centre at King's College Hospital in London, there has been a successful transition service for many years that has included staff from both the paediatric and adult diabetes teams, including psychologists, to allow for easier bridging of the gap between paediatric and adult services. Difficulties in family functioning may be associated with poorer glycaemic control (33).

There are many examples of good practice internationally, one such being the Joslin Diabetes Centre in Boston, where child mental health services, including a family intervention, have been embedded in paediatric services for many years (34). Recent work from Canada led by Tamara Spaic explored the role of a 'transition coordinator' in the transition from the paediatric to the young adult clinic. The transition coordinators were certified diabetes educators who provided transitional education and clinical support where appropriate. Patients randomised to the intervention arm demonstrated improved clinic attendance, reduced diabetes distress and improved satisfaction with care. However, these improvements were not seen in the 12 months following cessation of the intervention, raising concerns that the transition coordinator may be perceived as a 'Diabetes Mom', whereas the real goal is to foster independence and interdependence among young people (35). The D1 Now study, which is still at the pilot randomised controlled trial stage, is exploring a similar approach by using a support worker to help young adults (18–25 years of age) engage more with diabetes services (36). The complex intervention in the D1 Now study also incorporates a clinic-based tool that aims to measure diabetes distress and to enable discussion of the burden of living with type 1 diabetes (alongside more traditional measures of diabetes care, including HbA1c and risk of hypoglycaemia) during the clinic encounter (37). Preliminary qualitative data from the D1 Now cohort suggest that young people really value being asked about the burden of living with diabetes.

Liaison Endocrinologists

Liaison psychiatrists are psychiatrists that work in the acute hospital setting and deliver mental healthcare to people with acute physical healthcare needs. For example, they will often be involved in the care of people who have been admitted with DKA and who also have a depressive illness. The JBDS/RCPsych guidelines suggest that it may be worth considering a mirror of this model for inpatient mental health settings, where endocrinologists provide physical healthcare as a liaison diabetologist or liaison endocrinologist (2). There are some examples where this is already in place, where endocrinology provides inreach into mental health settings, such as the endocrinology inreach service to a medium secure setting in Hampshire, UK (2). This has been successful in providing timely management of diabetes in mental health settings.

Conclusion: Equity of Access to Physical Healthcare – Closing the Gap

Diabetes is common in mental health facilities and settings, where it is more common than in the general population. Diabetes as a cardiovascular risk factor contributes greatly to the mortality gap faced by people with SMI, and we must act to reduce this gap by optimising the detection and management of diabetes in these settings. Factors such as acuity of illness, lack of insight into both mental and physical health problems and practical difficulties in attending appointments, where present, may work against optimised diabetes management.

The key to delivering the best care for people with diabetes and comorbid mental disorders is collaboration and communication, and where this exists care is likely to be more effective. We have outlined some suggestions for how this can be achieved at an institutional level and also by individual clinicians and innovators. Any of the above points might be seen as quality improvement initiatives. Specific measures may be required to ensure that patients in these settings receive the usual standard of care.

References

1 Roberts E, Jones L, Blackman A, Dewhurst T, Matcham F, Kan C, et al. The prevalence of diabetes mellitus and abnormal glucose metabolism in the inpatient psychiatric setting: a systematic review and meta-analysis. *Gen Hosp Psychiatry*. 2017; 45: 76–84.

2 JBDS, RCPsych. *The Management of Diabetes in Adults and Children with Psychiatric Disorders in Inpatient Settings*. Joint British Diabetes Societies and Royal College of Psychiatrists, 2017.

3 NICE. *Type 2 Diabetes in Adults: Management [NG28]*. National Institute for Health and Care Excellence, 2015.

4   NICE. *Type 1 Diabetes in Adults: Diagnosis and Management [NG17]*. National Institute for Health and Care Excellence, 2015.

5   Taylor DM, Paton C, Kapur S. *The Maudsley Prescribing Guidelines in Psychiatry*. Wiley Blackwell, 2015.

6   ADA. Consensus development conference on antipsychotic drugs and obesity and diabetes. *Obes Res*. 2004; 12(2): 362–8.

7   Cohen D, Bogers JP, van Dijk D, Bakker B, Schulte PF. Beyond white blood cell monitoring: screening in the initial phase of clozapine therapy. *J Clin Psychiatry*. 2012; 73(10): 1307–12.

8   Morrato EH, Newcomer JW, Kamat S, Baser O, Harnett J, Cuffel B. Metabolic screening after the American Diabetes Association's consensus statement on antipsychotic drugs and diabetes. *Diabetes Care*. 2009; 32(6): 1037–42.

9   Holt RIG, Gossage-Worrall R, Hind D, Bradburn MJ, McCrone P, Morris T, et al. Structured lifestyle education for people with schizophrenia, schizoaffective disorder and first-episode psychosis (STEPWISE): randomised controlled trial. *Br J Psychiatry*. 2019; 214(2): 63–73.

10 Lowndes R. *Diabetes Care and Serious Mental Illness: An Institutional Ethnography*. Doctoral thesis. University of Toronto, 2012.

11 Hurley L, O'Donnell M, O'Caoimh R, Dinneen SF. Investigating the management of diabetes in nursing homes using a mixed methods approach. *Diabetes Res Clin Pract*. 2017; 127: 156–62.

12 Samara MT, Dold M, Gianatsi M, Nikolakopoulou A, Helfer B, Salanti G, et al. Efficacy, acceptability, and tolerability of antipsychotics in treatment-resistant schizophrenia: a network meta-analysis. *JAMA Psychiatry*. 2016; 73(3): 199–210.

13 Henderson DC, Cagliero E, Gray C, Nasrallah RA, Hayden DL, Schoenfeld DA, et al. Clozapine, diabetes mellitus, weight gain, and lipid abnormalities: a five-year naturalistic study. *Am J Psychiatry*. 2000; 157(6): 975–81.

14 de Silva VA, Suraweera C, Ratnatunga SS, Dayabandara M, Wanniarachchi N, Hanwella R. Metformin in prevention and treatment of antipsychotic induced weight gain: a systematic review and meta-analysis. *BMC Psychiatry*. 2016; 16 (1): 341.

15 Ellinger LK, Ipema HJ, Stachnik JM. Efficacy of metformin and topiramate in prevention and treatment of second-generation antipsychotic-induced weight gain. *Ann Pharmacother*. 2010; 44(4): 668–79.

16 Jiang WL, Cai DB, Yin F, Zhang L, Zhao XW, He J, et al. Adjunctive metformin for antipsychotic-induced dyslipidemia: a meta-analysis of randomized, double-blind, placebo-controlled trials. *Transl Psychiatry*. 2020; 10(1): 117.

17 Svensson CK, Larsen JR, Vedtofte L, Jakobsen MSL, Jespersen HR, Jakobsen MI, et al. One-year follow-up on liraglutide treatment for prediabetes and overweight/obesity in clozapine- or olanzapine-treated patients. *Acta Psychiatr Scand*. 2019; 139 (1): 26–36.

18 Larsen JR, Vedtofte L, Jakobsen MSL, Jespersen HR, Jakobsen MI, Svensson CK, et al. Effect of liraglutide treatment on prediabetes and overweight or obesity in clozapine- or olanzapine-treated patients with schizophrenia spectrum disorder: a randomized clinical trial. *JAMA Psychiatry*. 2017; 74(7): 719–28.

19 Pozzi M, Mazhar F, Peeters G, Vantaggiato C, Nobile M, Clementi E, et al. A systematic review of the antidepressant effects of glucagon-like peptide 1 (GLP-1) functional agonists: Further link between metabolism and psychopathology: Special Section on 'Translational and Neuroscience Studies in Affective Disorders'. Section Editor, Maria Nobile MD, PhD. This Section of JAD focuses on the relevance of translational and neuroscience studies in providing a better understanding of the neural basis of affective disorders. The main aim is to briefly summaries relevant research findings in clinical neuroscience with particular regards to specific innovative topics in mood and anxiety disorders.

J Affect Disord. 2019; 257: S0165-0327(19) 30593-2.

20 Gamble JM, Chibrikov E, Midodzi WK, Twells LK, Majumdar SR. Examining the risk of depression or self-harm associated with incretin-based therapies used to manage hyperglycaemia in patients with type 2 diabetes: a cohort study using the UK Clinical Practice Research Datalink. *BMJ Open.* 2018; 8(10): e023830.

21 Dixit TS, Sharma AN, Lucot JB, Elased KM. Antipsychotic-like effect of GLP-1 agonist liraglutide but not DPP-IV inhibitor sitagliptin in mouse model for psychosis. *Physiol Behav.* 2013; 114–115: 38–41.

22 Chowdhury TA, Wright R, Charlton M. Insulin for the uninitiated. *Clin Med (Lond).* 2014; 14(6): 623–9.

23 Southern Health NHS Foundation Trust. *Delegation of Medicines Administration to Non Registered Practitioners and Paid Carers by Registered Nurses in Integrated Community Services and Learning Disability.* Southern Health NHS Foundation Trust, 2019.

24 Gillespie H, Findlay White F, Kennedy N, Dornan T. *Enhancing Workplace Learning at the Transition into Practice. Lessons from a Pandemic.* Medical Education, 2020.

25 Teasdale SB, Samaras K, Wade T, Jarman R, Ward PB. A review of the nutritional challenges experienced by people living with severe mental illness: a role for dietitians in addressing physical health gaps. *J Hum Nutr Diet.* 2017; 30(5): 545–53.

26 Hunt K, Stiller K. Dietetic and educational interventions improve clinical outcomes of diabetic and obese clients with mental impairment. *Nutr Diet.* 2017; 74(3): 236–42.

27 Curtis J, Watkins A, Rosenbaum S, Teasdale S, Kalucy M, Samaras K, et al. Evaluating an individualized lifestyle and life skills intervention to prevent antipsychotic-induced weight gain in first-episode psychosis. *Early Interv Psychiatry.* 2016; 10(3): 267–76.

28 Whittemore R, Jaser S, Chao A, Jang M, Grey M. Psychological experience of

parents of children with type 1 diabetes: a systematic mixed-studies review. *Diabetes Educ.* 2012; 38(4): 562–79.

29 Polonsky WH, Anderson BJ, Lohrer PA, Welch G, Jacobson AM, Aponte JE, et al. Assessment of diabetes-related distress. *Diabetes Care.* 1995; 18(6): 754–60.

30 Hagger V, Hendrieckx C, Sturt J, Skinner TC, Speight J. Diabetes distress among adolescents with type 1 diabetes: a systematic review. *Curr Diab Rep.* 2016; 16 (1): 9.

31 Huxley RR, Peters SA, Mishra GD, Woodward M. Risk of all-cause mortality and vascular events in women versus men with type 1 diabetes: a systematic review and meta-analysis. *Lancet Diabetes Endocrinol.* 2015; 3(3): 198–206.

32 Eiser C, Johnson B, Brierley S, Ayling K, Young V, Bottrell K, et al. Using the Medical Research Council framework to develop a complex intervention to improve delivery of care for young people with type 1 diabetes. *Diabet Med.* 2013; 30(6): e223–8.

33 Jacobson AM, Hauser ST, Lavori P, Willett JB, Cole CF, Wolfsdorf JI, et al. Family environment and glycemic control: a four-year prospective study of children and adolescents with insulin-dependent diabetes mellitus. *Psychosom Med.* 1994; 56 (5): 401–9.

34 Laffel LM, Vangsness L, Connell A, Goebel-Fabbri A, Butler D, Anderson BJ. Impact of ambulatory, family-focused teamwork intervention on glycemic control in youth with type 1 diabetes. *J Pediatr.* 2003; 142(4): 409–16.

35 Spaic T, Robinson T, Goldbloom E, Gallego P, Hramiak I, Lawson ML, et al. Closing the gap: results of the multicenter canadian randomized controlled trial of structured transition in young adults with type 1 diabetes. *Diabetes Care.* 2019; 42(6): 1018–26.

36 Casey B, Byrne M, Casey D, Gillespie P, Hobbins A, Newell J, et al. Improving outcomes among young adults with type 1 diabetes: the D1 Now randomised pilot

study protocol. *Diabetic Med.* 2020; 37(9): 1590–604.

37 Todd PJ, Edwards F, Spratling L, Patel NH, Amiel SA, Sturt J, et al. Evaluating the relationships of hypoglycaemia and HbA1c with screening-detected diabetes distress in type 1 diabetes. *Endocrinol Diabetes Metab.* 2018; 1(1): e00003.

Index